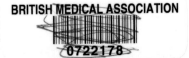

"To my wife, Angela, for her enlightening encouragement and endless humor."
C.P.H.

"To my wife and child who have always supported and inspired me."
A.B.B.

"To my loving wife Lori for all her support."
J.M.P.

"My thanks and love to my family—King, Lauren, Anne, Chip, and Katherine."
W.J.B.

Visual Diagnosis in Emergency and Critical Care Medicine

EDITED BY

Christopher P. Holstege | MD, FACEP, FAAEM, FACMT
Director, Division of Medical Toxicology
Medical Director, Blue Ridge Poison Center
Associate Professor, Departments of Emergency Medicine and Pediatrics
University of Virginia
Charlottesville
Virginia

Alexander B. Baer | MD
Associate Medical Director, Blue Ridge Poison Center
Clinical Assistant Professor, Department of Emergency Medicine
University of Virginia
Charlottesville
Virginia

Jesse M. Pines | MD, MBA, FAAEM
Lecturer, Department of Emergency Medicine
Center for Clinical Epidemiology and Biostatistics
University of Pennsylvania School of Medicine
Philadelphia
Pennsylvania

William J. Brady | MD, FACEP, FAAEM
Vice Chair, Department of Emergency Medicine
Professor, Department of Emergency Medicine and Internal Medicine
University of Virginia
Charlottesville
Virginia

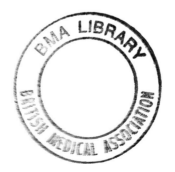

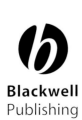

Blackwell
Publishing

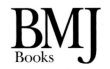

BMJ
Books

© 2006 by Blackwell Publishing Ltd
BMJ Books is an imprint of the BMJ Publishing Group Limited, used under licence

Blackwell Publishing, Inc., 350 Main Street, Malden, Massachusetts 02148-5020, USA
Blackwell Publishing Ltd, 9600 Garsington Road, Oxford OX4 2DQ, UK
Blackwell Publishing Asia Pty Ltd, 550 Swanston Street, Carlton, Victoria 3053, Australia

The right of the author to be identified as the author of this work has been asserted in
accordance with the Copyright, Designs and Patents Act 1988.

First published 2006

1 2006

Library of Congress Cataloging-in-Publication Data
Visual diagnosis in emergency and critical care medicine/edited by Christopher P.
Holstege . . . [et al.].
        p. ; cm.
    Includes bibliographical references and index.
    ISBN-13: 978-1-4051-3491-0 (alk. paper)
    ISBN-10: 1-4051-3491-7 (alk. paper)
   1. Emergency medical services—Case studies. 2. Critical care medicine—Case studies.
3. Diagnosis. I. Holstege, Christopher P.
      [DNLM: 1. Emergency Medicine—Case Reports. 2. Emergency Medicine—Examination
Questions. 3. Critical Care—Case Reports. 4. Critical Care—Examination Questions.
5. Diagnosis—Case Reports. 6. Diagnosis—Examination Questions. WB 18.2 V834 2007]

      RA645.5.V57 2007
      362.18—dc22   2006022486

ISBN-13: 978-1-4051-3491-0
ISBN-10: 1-4051-3491-7

A catalogue record for this title is available from the British Library

Set in 9/12 pt Meridien by Charon Tec Ltd (A Macmillan Company), Chennai, India
www.charontec.com
Printed and bound in Singapore by COS Printers Pte Ltd

Commissioning Editor: Mary Banks
Editorial Assistant: Victoria Pittman
Development Editor: Nick Morgan
Production Controller: Debbie Wyer

For further information on Blackwell Publishing, visit our website:
http://www.blackwellpublishing.com

The publisher's policy is to use permanent paper from mills that operate a sustainable forestry
policy, and which has been manufactured from pulp processed using acid-free and elementary
chlorine-free practices. Furthermore, the publisher ensures that the text paper and cover board
used have met acceptable environmental accreditation standards.

Contents

List of contributors

Alexander B. Baer, MD
Associate Medical Director, Blue Ridge Poison Center, and Clinical Assistant Professor, Department of Emergency Medicine, University of Virginia, PO Box 800774, Charlottesville, VA 22908-0774

Roger A. Band, MD
Assistant Professor, Department of Emergency Medicine, University of Pennsylvania School of Medicine, 3400 Spruce Street, Philadelphia, PA 19104

Kevin L. Barlotta, MD
Emergency Medicine Resident, Department of Emergency Medicine, University of Virginia, PO Box 800774, Charlottesville, VA 22908-0774

Mara Becker, MD
Fellow, Pediatric Rheumatology, Alfred I. duPont Hospital for Children, 1600 Rockland Road, Wilmington, DE 19803

Chris S. Bergstrom, MD
Fellow, Vitreoretinal Surgery, Department of Ophthalmology, Emory University, 201 Dowman Drive, Atlanta, GA 30322

Christopher T. Bowe, MD
Associate Residency Director, Emergency Medicine Department, Maine Medical Center, 22 Bramhall Street, Portland, ME 04102

William J. Brady, MD, FACEP, FAAEM
Vice Chair, Department of Emergency Medicine, and Professor, Department of Emergency Medicine and Internal Medicine, University of Virginia, PO Box 800669, Charlottesville, VA 22908-0699

Craig S. Brummer, MD
Attending Physician, Kennestone Hospital, 4016 Benell Court, Smyrna, GA 30082

Brendan E. Carr, MD, MA
Instructor, Department of Emergency Medicine, and Fellow, Division of Trauma and Surgical Critical Care, Department of Surgery, University of Pennsylvania School of Medicine, 3400 Spruce Street, Philadelphia, PA 19104

Maureen Chase, MD
Instructor and Research Fellow, Department of Emergency Medicine, University of Pennsylvania School of Medicine, 3400 Spruce Street, Philadelphia, PA 19104

Esther H. Chen, MD
Assistant Professor, Department of Emergency Medicine, University of Pennsylvania School of Medicine, 3400 Spruce Street, Philadelphia, PA 19104

Anthony J. Dean, MD
Director, Emergency Ultrasound, and Assistant Professor, Department of Emergency Medicine, University of Pennsylvania School of Medicine, 3400 Spruce Street, Philadelphia, PA 19104

David L. Eldridge, MD
Assistant Professor, Department of Pediatrics, Brody School of Medicine, East Carolina University, 600 Moye Boulevard, Greenville, NC 27834

Worth W. Everett, MD
Assistant Professor, Department of Emergency Medicine, University of Pennsylvania School of Medicine, 3400 Spruce Street, Philadelphia, PA 19104

David F. Gaieski, MD
Co-Director, Early Goal Directed Therapy Program, and Assistant Professor, Department of Emergency Medicine, University of Pennsylvania School of Medicine, 3400 Spruce Street, Philadelphia, PA 19104

Munish Goyal, MD
Co-Director, Early Goal Directed Therapy Program, and Assistant Professor, Department of Emergency Medicine, University of Pennsylvania School of Medicine, 3400 Spruce Street, Philadelphia, PA 19104

Christopher P. Holstege, MD, FACEP, FAAEM, FACMT
Director, Division of Medical Toxicology, Medical Director, Blue Ridge Poison Center, and Associate Professor, Departments of Emergency Medicine and Pediatrics, University of Virginia, PO Box 800774, Charlottesville, VA 22908-0774

Andrew L. Homer
Medical Student, University of Virginia School of Medicine, PO Box 800774, Charlottesville, VA 22908-0774

David A. Kasper, MBA
Philadelphia College of Osteopathic Medicine, c/o Kenneth Katz, MD, Department of Dermatology, University of Pennsylvania School of Medicine, 3600 Spruce Street, Philadelphia, PA 19104

Kenneth A. Katz, MD, MSc
Instructor and NRSA Postdoctoral Fellow, Department of Dermatology, University of Pennsylvania School of Medicine, 3600 Spruce Street, Philadelphia, PA 19104

Allyson Kreshak, MD
Resident Physician, Department of Emergency Medicine, University of Pennsylvania School of Medicine, c/o Jesse M. Pines, 3400 Spruce Street, Philadelphia, PA 19104

Bon S. Ku, MD
Instructor and Ultrasound Fellow, Department of Emergency Medicine, University of Pennsylvania School of Medicine, 3400 Spruce Street, Philadelphia, PA 19104

Hoi Lee, MD
Resident Physician, Department of Emergency Medicine, University of Pennsylvania School of Medicine, 3400 Spruce Street, Philadelphia, PA 19104

Rex Mathew, MD
Assistant Professor, Department of Emergency Medicine, Thomas Jefferson University, 1020 Walnut Street, Philadelphia, PA 19107

Angela M. Mills, MD
Assistant Professor, Department of Emergency Medicine, University of Pennsylvania School of Medicine, 3400 Spruce Street, Philadelphia, PA 19104

Andrea L. Neimann, MD
Department of Dermatology, University of Pennsylvania School of Medicine, c/o Jesse M. Pines, 3400 Spruce Street, Philadelphia, PA 19104

Susan A. O'Malley, MD
Associate Attending, Brookhaven Memorial Hospital Medical Center, 101 Hospital Road, Patchogue, NY 11772

Andrew D. Perron, MD
Residency Director, Department of Emergency Medicine, 22 Bramhall Street, Main Medical Center, Portland, ME 04102

Jesse M. Pines, MD, MBA, FAAEM
Lecturer, Department of Emergency Medicine, Center for Clinical Epidemiology and Biostatistics, University of Pennsylvania School of Medicine, 3400 Spruce Street, Philadelphia, PA 19104

Jane M. Prosser, MD
Resident Physician, Department of Emergency Medicine, University of Pennsylvania School of Medicine, 3400 Spruce Street, Philadelphia, PA 19104

Tracy H. Reilly, MD
Fellow, Medical Toxicology, Department of Emergency Medicine, University of Virginia, PO Box 800774, Charlottesville, VA 22908-0774

Joseph Robson, MD
Chief Resident Physician, Department of Emergency Medicine, University of Pennsylvania School of Medicine, 3400 Spruce Street, Philadelphia, PA 19104

Adam K. Rowden, DO
Fellow, Medical Toxicology, Department of Emergency Medicine, University of Virginia, PO Box 800774, Charlottesville, VA 22908-0774

Aradhna Saxena, MD
Resident, Department of Dermatology and Cutaneous Biology, Thomas Jefferson University Hospital, 833 Chestnut Street, Philadelphia, PA 19107

Suzanne M. Shepherd, MD, DTM&H
Associate Professor, Department of Emergency Medicine, and Director of Education and Research, PENN Travel Medicine, University of Pennsylvania School of Medicine, 3400 Spruce Street, Philadelphia, PA 19104

William H. Shoff, MD, DTM&H
Associate Professor, Department of Emergency Medicine, and Director, PENN Travel Medicine, University of Pennsylvania School of Medicine, 3400 Spruce Street, Philadelphia, PA 19104

Daniel K. Vining, MD
Resident Physician, Department of Emergency Medicine, University of Pennsylvania School of Medicine, 3400 Spruce Street, Philadelphia, PA 19104

Edward G. Walsh, MD
Emergency Medicine Resident, Department of Emergency Medicine, University of Virginia, PO Box 800774, Charlottesville, VA 22908-0774

Sarah G. Winters, MD
Fellow, Division of General Pediatrics, Children's Hospital of Philadelphia, c/o Brendan Carr, MD, 3400 Spruce Street, Philadelphia, PA 19104

Foreword

Emergency physicians often have a knack for making rapid diagnoses and initiating needed treatments quickly. Developing one's ability to blend visual, historical and physical clues is generally based upon a combination of understanding basic pathophysiological mechanisms, identifying important historical and physical findings known to be associated with these pathophysiological mechanisms, and re-experiencing imprinted visual cues from prior cases. This visual diagnosis book, written by Holstege, Baer, Pines and Brady, takes advantage of all these features in an effort to serve as a valuable teaching tool for the physician or medical student seeking to improve their ability to rapidly diagnose important clinical conditions that may present to virtually any emergency department.

The cases are not arranged by body system or by pathophysiological mechanisms (e.g., trauma, infectious disease, etc). Rather, they are presented similar to cases appearing in the emergency department. Thus, they appear in no particular order or sequence. Children are interspersed with adults and injuries with medical conditions.

Each case is presented as an unknown along with a graphic illustration, brief case presentation, and management decision. The photos and line drawings are crisp and generally well demonstrate the patient's abnormality, although some presentations may be subtle to the uninitiated. The answers provided later in the book are much richer than would be anticipated for a case presentation text. The discussions and supplemental illustrations create the impression that you have a seasoned emergency physician in the room who is walking you through the basic pathophysiological mechanisms and then clarifying the visual clues and their clinical significance. This detail gives you the confidence that you can recognize and respond appropriately were you to re-experience these case presentations in the future.

As a seasoned clinician, I eagerly read the case presentations first to verify my own rapid diagnostic skills and secondarily to determine if the authors would approach the problem as I would or if they would make different interventional recommendations. Although I am pleased that my interpretations were highly correlated with those of the authors, I found the richness of their discussion valuable for refreshing my understanding of the mechanisms behind the illness associated with each image.

I anticipate that learners (whether novices or seasoned continued learners like myself) will appreciate what this book has to offer. It is fun and easy to pick up and begin the learning. Unfortunately, it is sometimes hard to put down for these same reasons. I anticipate keeping this text handy to reinforce key teaching points with medical students and residents. Others may find the text extremely valuable for preparing for the visual image portion of the emergency medicine written board examination. Those of us who have been away from our residency for some time will enjoy the text as a stimulus leading us to re-experience visual clues on conditions we simply don't want to miss as clinicians.

I anticipate that this text will be popular and eventually lead to subsequent "Visual Diagnosis" volumes. Our students and practitioners will be pleased to see these as well.

Jerris R. Hedges, MD, MS
Professor of Emergency Medicine
Vice Dean, School of Medicine
Oregon Health & Sciences University

Preface

The acute care practitioner faces numerous challenges in the approach to the critically ill or injured patient. Clearly, the history of the event is a vital portion of the evaluation, providing the "answer" to the clinical situation in many instances. The physical examination and the results of various diagnostic investigations, however, are also essential components of the medical evaluation. In fact, the examination, the electrocardiogram, and the radiograph provide the clinician with either the diagnosis or important information which will lead to the diagnosis. The rash of erythema multiforme, the electrocardiogram in pronounced hyperkalemia, the radiograph in carpometacarpal dislocation are all presentations where a single "clinical image" provides the diagnosis or a substantial clue to the diagnosis – with appropriate therapy soon to follow. Bedside clinical diagnosis, based upon specific clinical images, is a vital skill for the acute care practitioner.

The purpose of this book is to provide some of those visual diagnostic clues that might be encountered in acute care scenarios. In Part 1, each visual cue is associated with an actual case and a multiple choice question. The correct answer and a focused discussion then follow in Part 2. In academic practice, utilizing a visual cue with an associated case presentation and a multiple choice question is a highly effective teaching method. In clinical practice, the use of case-based scenarios is a popular, effective means of self-education. This enables the teacher or the student to discuss the disease, and importantly the diagnosis and management. We have attempted to capture this teaching style within the context of this book. Whether you are an experienced clinician in private practice, an academician engaged in teaching, a resident or student in training looking to prepare for tests, we hope this book will provide you with further experience to excel as a practitioner in the field of medicine.

Christopher P. Holstege
Alexander B. Baer
Jesse M. Pines
William J. Brady

Illustration credits

1 **Poison Ivy.** Case: Christopher P. Holstege; Figs 1 and 2: Christopher P. Holstege

2 **Digoxin Toxicity.** Case: Christopher P. Holstege

3 **Angle Closure Glaucoma.** Case: Chris S. Bergstrom

4 **Boxer's Fracture.** Case: Alexander B. Baer; Fig. 1: Alexander B. Baer

5 **Abdominal Aortic Aneurysm.** Case: Anthony J. Dean; Figs 1 and 2: Anthony J. Dean

6 **Coining.** Case: Edward T. Dickinson

7 **Perilunate dislocation.** Case: Alexander B. Baer; Fig. 1: Alexander B. Baer

8 **Drug Hypersensitivity Reaction.** Case: Christopher P. Holstege; Figs 1 and 2: Christopher P. Holstege

9 **Egyptian with Hemolysis.** Case: William H. Shoff

10 **Retropharyngeal Abscess.** Case: Alexander B. Baer

11 **Hyperkalemia.** Case: William J. Brady; Figs 1 and 2: William J. Brady

12 **Conjunctivitis.** Case: Chris S. Bergstrom

13 **Buckle Fracture.** Case: Alexander B. Baer; Fig. 1: Alexander B. Baer

14 **Cholecystitis.** Case: Anthony J. Dean; Fig. 1: Anthony J. Dean

15 **Smoke Inhalation.** Case: Christopher P. Holstege; Fig. 1: Christopher P. Holstege

16 **Lumbar Wedge Fracture.** Case: Alexander B. Baer; Fig. 1: Alexander B. Baer

17 **Snakebite.** Case: Alexander B. Baer; Fig. 1: Christopher P. Holstege

18 **Submandibular Abscess.** Case: Alexander B. Baer

19 **Sail Sign.** Case: Alexander B. Baer; Fig. 1: Alexander B. Baer

20 **SVC Syndrome.** Case: Alexander B. Baer

21 **Inferoposterior RV AMI.** Case: William J. Brady; Fig. 1: William J. Brady

22 **Corneal Abrasion.** Case: Chris S. Bergstrom

23 **Button Battery.** Case: Sarah G. Winters; Figs 1–4: Sarah G. Winters

24 **Ectopic.** Case: Anthony J. Dean; Figs 1 and 2: Anthony J. Dean

25 **Syphilis.** Case: William D. James

26 **Lumbar Teardrop Fracture.** Case: Alexander B. Baer; Fig. 1: Alexander B. Baer

27 **Sporotrichosis.** Case: Steve Larson

28 **Tuberculosis Adenitis.** Case: William H. Shoff

29 **Salter–Harris Fracture.** Case: William J. Brady; Figs 1 and 2: William J. Brady

30 **Raccoon Eyes.** Case: Alexander B. Baer

31 **LBBB AMI.** Case: William J. Brady; Fig. 1: William J. Brady

32 **Corneal Ulcer.** Case: Chris S. Bergstrom

33 **Calcaneus Fracture.** Case: Alexander B. Baer; Fig. 1: Alexander B. Baer

34 **Fast Exam.** Case: Anthony J. Dean; Figs 1 and 2: Anthony J. Dean

35 **Skin Popping.** Case: Alexander B. Baer; Figs 1–3: Alexander B. Baer; Fig. 4: Christopher P. Holstege

36 **Lumbar Pars Defect.** Case: Christopher P. Holstege; Fig. 1: Christopher P. Holstege

37 **Rhabdomyolysis.** Case: Christopher P. Holstege; Fig. 1: Christopher P. Holstege

38 **Long QT Syndrome.** Case: William J. Brady

39 **Scaphoid Fracture.** Case: Alexander B. Baer; Figs 1 and 2: Alexander B. Baer

40 **Pyoderma Gangrenosum.** Case: Kenneth A. Katz

41 **LVH.** Case: William J. Brady; Fig. 1: William J. Brady

42 **Eye Chemical Injury.** Case: Chris S. Bergstrom

43 **Carpometacarpal Dislocation.** Case: Alexander B. Baer; Fig. 1: Alexander B. Baer

44 **Pericardial Tamponade.** Case: Anthony J. Dean; Figs 1–4: Anthony J. Dean

45 **Penetrating Neck Injury.** Case: Alexander B. Baer

46 **Lisfranc Fracture.** Case: Alexander B. Baer

47 **Erythema Multiforme.** Case: Brendan E. Carr

48 **Frostbite.** Case: Alexander B. Baer

49 **Herbal Aconitine.** Case: Christopher P. Holstege

50 **Sentinel Loop.** Case: Alexander B. Baer

51 **Gas Gangrene.** Case: Alexander B. Baer

52 **Pericarditis.** Case: William J. Brady

53 **Eyelid Laceration.** Case: Chris S. Bergstrom

54 **Monteggia.** Case: Alexander B. Baer; Fig. 1: Alexander B. Baer

55 **Avascular Necrosis.** Case: Alexander B. Baer

56 **Herpes Zoster.** Case: Alexander B. Baer

57 **Lead Paint Chips.** Case: Christopher P. Holstege; Fig. 1: Christopher P. Holstege

58 **Hydrofluoric Acid.** Case: Christopher P. Holstege

59 **HSP.** Case: Mara Becker

60 **Pneumoperitoneum.** Case: Munish Goyal

61 **Injection Injury.** Case: Alexander B. Baer; Fig. 1: Alexander B. Baer

62 **ST Elevation BER.** Case: William J. Brady; Fig. 1: William J. Brady

63 **Globe Rupture.** Case: Chris S. Bergstrom

64 **Cauda Equina Syndrome.** Case: Alexander B. Baer; Fig. 1: Alexander B. Baer

Part 1 | Case Presentations and Questions

Case 1 | **Rash following brush fire**

Christopher P. Holstege, MD

Case presentation: A 9-year-old male presents to the emergency department with facial pain, erythema, and swelling. He was in his normal state of health until this morning when he awoke from sleep and noted a diffuse rash over

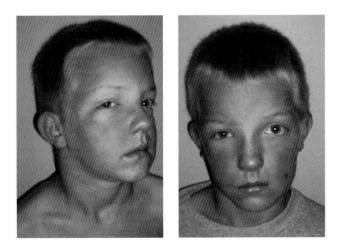

his face with a marked burning sensation in the region of the rash. It has progressed through the day and involves only his face and neck and stops at his shirt neckline. He has had no fevers and his immunizations are up to date. He denies any other complaints. His best friend also awoke with the same rash. The previous day, while playing on the school playground, they watched a neighboring farm burning brush. Smoke from the fire blew over the area where they were watching. His facial examination is pictured as shown.

Question: The rash is due to:
A Type 1 allergic reaction
B Type 4 allergic reaction
C Roseola
D Rubella (German measles)
E Rubeola (measles)

See page 67 for Answer, Diagnosis, and Discussion.

Case 2 | **Herbalist with bradycardia and vision changes**

William J. Brady, MD

Case presentation: A 33-year-old female herbalist presents to the emergency department with a complaint of weakness and yellow discoloration of her vision. She recently grew the plant pictured at right and is ingesting it as an herbal remedy in an attempt to alleviate menstrual cramps.

On arrival, the patient is alert and oriented. Her initial vital signs are blood pressure 110/60 mmHg, pulse 88 beats/minute, respirations 28 breaths/minute. The rest of her examination is unremarkable. An initial 12-lead electrocardiogram (ECG) demonstrates a normal sinus rhythm with multiple premature ventricular contractions (PVC).

Her electrolyte results returned from the laboratory demonstrating marked hyperkalemia. She subsequently developed progressive bradycardia (see rhythm strip on the next page) over the ensuing 60 minutes.

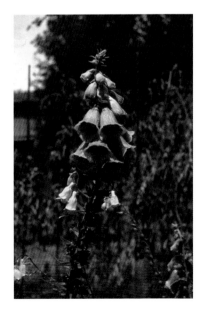

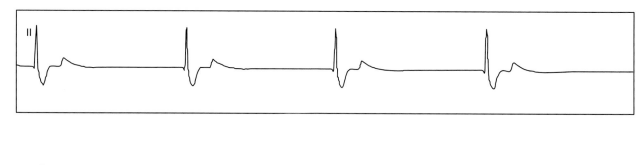

Question: Which of the following would be appropriate in the management of this patient?
A Digoxin-specific Fab fragments
B Physostigmine
C Naloxone
D Flumazenil
E Amiodarone

See page 67 for Answer, Diagnosis, and Discussion.

Case 3 | **Acute eye pain and blurred vision in an elderly female**

Chris S. Bergstrom, MD & Alexander B. Baer, MD

Case presentation: A 68-year-old female with no significant past medical history presents to the emergency department complaining of pain, blurred vision, and colored halos around lights in her left eye. She states that her visual symptoms started acutely along with associated nausea, vomiting, and a frontal headache.

On physical examination the visual acuity is 20/30 in the right eye and 20/100 in the left. Pupillary exam reveals a sluggish, mid-dilated pupil in the left eye as noted in the picture. Slit lamp examination of the left eye shows conjunctival injection with a cloudy cornea. The anterior chamber is shallow and the iris detail is blurred. Palpation of the globes through closed lids demonstrates a normal tension in the right eye and a firm, tense left eye. Intraocular pressures are measured and reveal 15 mmHg in the right eye and 58 mmHg in the left.

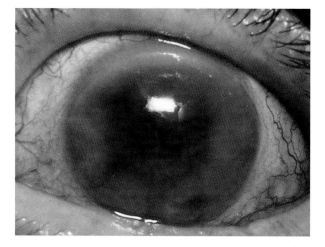

Question: Which of the following agents would be appropriate to administer to this patient?
A Subcutaneous epinephrine
B Topical atropine
C Topical timolol
D Intravenous atropine
E Topical phenylephrine

See page 68 for Answer, Diagnosis, and Discussion.

Case 4 | **Suspicious hand pain**

Rex Mathew, MD

Case presentation: A 38-year-old man presents to the emergency department on a Saturday night with a right hand injury. He states that he simply bumped his hand on a bar stool. On exam, the skin is intact over the fist; there is swelling over the dorsum of the hand and tenderness over his right 5th metacarpal; the motor, sensory, and vascular exams are normal. An X-ray is obtained.

Question: What is the next most appropriate management strategy at this time?
A Reassure the patient that there is no fracture and discharge him with analgesics and ice
B Admit the patient for emergent orthopedic surgical repair
C Splint the patient and discharge with orthopedic referral
D Admit the patient for intravenous antibiotics given the almost certain chance that this represents a fight bite
E Admit the patient for rheumatologic evaluation

See page 69 for Answer, Diagnosis, and Discussion.

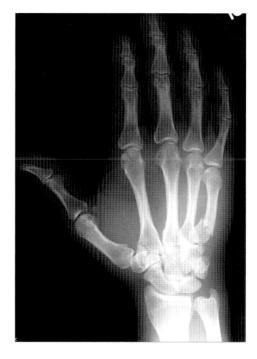

Case 5 | **An elderly man with flank pain**

Daniel K. Vining, MD & Anthony J. Dean, MD

Case presentation: A 73-year-old man with a history of obesity, hypertension, and cigarette smoking presents to the emergency department after a syncopal episode. He complains of mild left-sided back and flank pain. He has a blood pressure of 118/94 mmHg, pulse of 96 beats/minute, and respirations of 20 breaths/minute. The physical exam is significant only for mild diffuse abdominal discomfort to palpation with left back and flank tenderness to percussion. His urinalysis is normal. An ultrasound is performed. The image on the left shows a sagittal view of the aorta and the image on the right shows a transverse view of the aorta at the level of the renal veins.

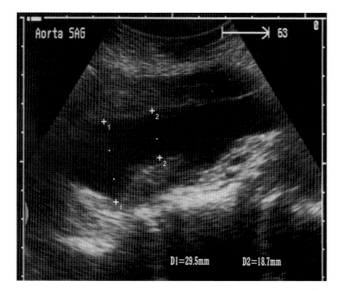

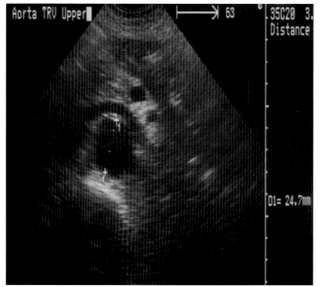

Question: Which of the following is true?

A The aorta imaged here has a normal diameter. This reduces the likelihood of abdominal aortic aneurysm (AAA) to less than 90%.

B The patient has an AAA. If no intra-abdominal free fluid is found in the abdomen, acute aortic aneurysm rupture is excluded from the differential diagnosis.

C The patient has an AAA. Immediate surgical consultation and operative intervention are needed.

D The patient has an AAA. Since the patient is comfortable and hemodynamically stable, he should be admitted for in-patient observation and further evaluation and imaging.

E The aorta imaged here shows significant stenosis. Doppler flow analysis or angiography is needed to identify whether this is the cause of the patient's acute symptoms.

See page 69 for Answer, Diagnosis, and Discussion.

Case 6 | An immigrant child with skin lesions

Roger A. Band, MD

Case presentation: A 14-year-old Vietnamese child presents accompanied by his grandmother, complaining of a non-productive cough, rhinorrhea, and low-grade fever to 100.2°F. The grandmother speaks little English, but once the mother arrives, she is able to give you the remaining history; specifically she denies any behavioral changes, trauma, or complaints of abdominal pain or arthralgias. On exam, the child appears generally well, with the exception of signs consistent with a viral upper respiratory tract infection, and the impressive lesions on his trunk pictured.

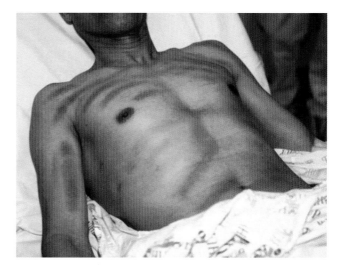

Question: What is the next most appropriate management strategy at this time?

A Give the child's mother appropriate return precautions and follow-up instructions, and reassure her that his upper respiratory tract complaints typically resolve in 2–3 days

B Order a CBC, blood culture, and urinalysis

C Call social work and child protective services

D Order a skeletal survey

E Discharge home with an antibiotic cream to be applied to the skin lesions

See page 70 for Answer, Diagnosis, and Discussion.

Case 7 | Wrist pain following a fall

Rex Mathew, MD

Case presentation: A 21-year-old man complains of left wrist pain after falling from a 5-foot ladder onto his left hand. On exam, there is swelling and tenderness over his wrist and exam is limited due to pain over the dorsum of his hand; the motor function is strong, and the sensory and vascular exams are otherwise normal. The wrist radiographs are noted as shown in the picture.

Question: What is the most likely injury?
A Scaphoid fracture
B Lunate dislocation
C Perilunate dislocation
D No fracture or dislocation; normal X-ray
E 5th metacarpal fracture

See page 71 for Answer, Diagnosis, and Discussion.

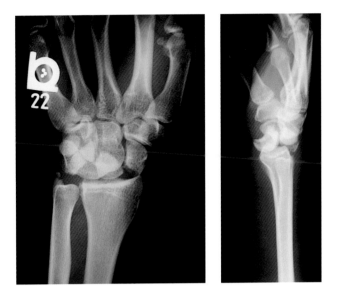

Case 8 | **Rash in a child with epilepsy**

Alexander B. Baer, MD & Christopher P. Holstege, MD

Case presentation: A 3-year-old female with a history of epilepsy and taking phenytoin presents to the emergency department with a rapidly progressing, painful rash, inability to swallow secretions, and difficulty breathing. The rash began 5 days previously, at which time her mother noted mild skin tenderness, low-grade fever, anorexia, and malaise. The child also complained of headache and developed diarrhea. She had been seen previously by three different health care providers over the past 5 days; all diagnosed her with a viral exanthema. When the child's mother awoke on the morning of arrival to the emergency department, she found her child with marked progression of the rash pictured at right that now involves her mucus membranes diffusely. In the emergency department, her vitals are as follows: blood pressure 67/34 mmHg, pulse 160 beats/minute, respirations 38 breaths/minute, and temperature 38.5°C. She is intubated and pictured at right. Her laboratory studies demonstrate that she has both renal and hepatic dysfunction.

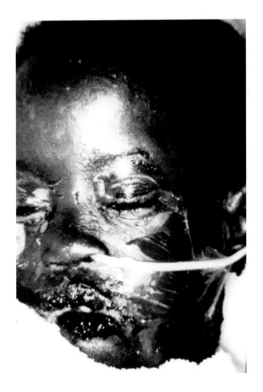

Question: Which of the following is correct regarding this child's condition?
A This child would be expected to have a positive Nikolsky's sign
B If this child had been started on antibiotics earlier, she would never have required intubation
C With proper treatment, this child's chances of survival are greater than 90%
D This is a primary dermatologic condition, with other organ involvement not expected
E She should be restarted on her phenytoin to avoid seizure complications

See page 72 for Answer, Diagnosis, and Discussion.

Case 9 | **Dark urine in an immigrant**

Suzanne M. Shepherd, MD, Susan A. O'Malley, MD & William H. Shoff, MD

Case presentation: A 38-year-old Egyptian male complains of progressive fatigue, skin and eye yellowing, crampy abdominal and low back pain, and darker urine over the past 2 days. He denies similar previous episodes. He notes no recent travel and no use of prescriptions, illicit drugs or herbal medicines. He denies alcohol ingestion, raw or tainted foods. He ate baked fish and lightly boiled broad beans approximately 16 hours prior to the onset of illness. Vital signs are remarkable only for a pulse of 108 beats/minute. Conjunctiva are pictured below; abdominal exam reveals mild diffuse tenderness. The spun urine is pictured below.

Question: Which of the following tests would be the most appropriate next step in his evaluation?
A Non-contrast computerized tomography (CT) scan to evaluate for nephrolithiasis
B Urine microscopy and peripheral blood smear
C Emergent endoscopic retrograde cholangiopancreatography
D Ultrasound of the gallbladder
E Chest and abdominal flat plate X-ray

See page 73 for Answer, Diagnosis, and Discussion.

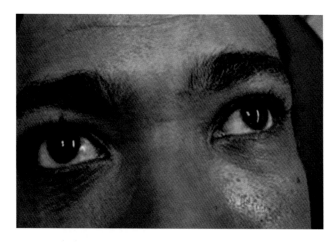

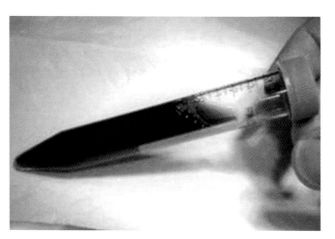

Case 10 | **Fever and drooling in a child**

Sarah G. Winters, MD & Brendan E. Carr, MD

Case presentation: An 18-month-old female presents with 2 days of fever and irritability. On the day of arrival to the emergency department, her mother reports the child has developed new onset of drooling and decreased oral intake. Her past medical history is unremarkable. On physical examination, she is febrile, ill appearing, and has neck stiffness. The following soft tissue lateral of the neck X-ray is obtained.

Question: What is the next most appropriate management strategy at this time?
A Discharge to home with supportive care
B Discharge to home with oral antibiotics
C Admit for intravenous antibiotics and surgical consultation
D Emergent intubation
E Cricothyroidotomy

See page 73 for Answer, Diagnosis, and Discussion.

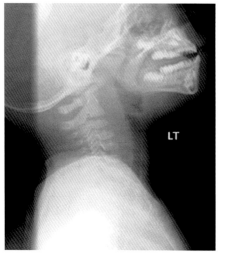

Case 11 | **Altered mental status with an abnormal electrocardiogram**

William J. Brady, MD

Case presentation: A 36-year-old female presented to the emergency department via private automobile with lethargy and weakness. Her past medical history and any further details regarding the current history of present illness were unavailable. On examination, the patient was lethargic but arousable; vitals signs were: blood pressure 100/70 mmHg, pulse 75 beats/minute, and respirations 16/minute. The remainder of the examination was unremarkable except for an apparent dialysis shunt in the left upper extremity. The electrocardiogram (ECG) is seen below.

Question: In this patient, the most likely diagnosis of this rhythm disturbance is:
A Ventricular tachycardia
B Idoventricular rhythm
C Junctional rhythm with bundle branch block
D Sinoventricular rhythm
E Normal sinus rhythm

See page 74 for Answer, Diagnosis, and Discussion.

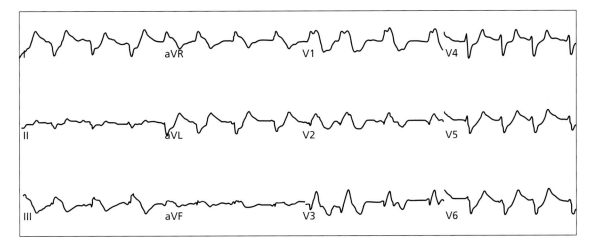

Case 12 | **Purulent eye discharge in an adult**

Chris S. Bergstrom, MD & Alexander B. Baer, MD

Case presentation: A 32-year-old male is seen in the emergency department complaining of left eye pain and ocular discharge. On physical examination, the visual acuity is mildly decreased to 20/30 in the left eye. Pupil examination is normal. There is a thick, copious, purulent discharge present from the left eye as noted in the figure. The conjunctiva is injected and chemotic but the cornea is clear.

Question: What is the appropriate treatment for this form of conjunctivitis?
A Topical acyclovir
B Topical erythromycin
C Intravenous ceftriaxone and topical ciprofloxacin
D Topical prednisolone
E Topical homatropine

See page 76 for Answer, Diagnosis, and Discussion.

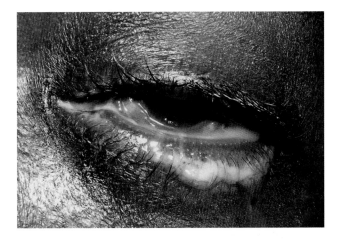

Case 13 | **Wrist pain in a young child**

Craig S. Brummer, MD

Case presentation: An 8-year-old boy fell onto his left outstretched arm after tripping on a sidewalk 2 days prior to arrival. He complains of ipsilateral wrist pain that worsens with movement. On exam, the child is holding a painful, minimally swollen left wrist. His motor, sensory, and vascular exams are normal, but he does have mild tenderness to palpation over his left lateral wrist. An X-ray is obtained and noted (see figure).

Question: Which management strategy is the most appropriate for this patient?
A Discharge home with no outpatient follow-up necessary
B Hematoma block with closed reduction
C Hospital admission with traction
D Emergent orthopedic surgical intervention
E Wrist immobilization and analgesic therapy

See page 76 for Answer, Diagnosis, and Discussion.

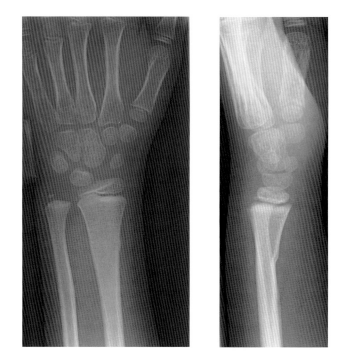

Case 14 | **Postprandial abdominal pain**

Anthony J. Dean, MD

Case presentation: A 32-year-old female presents with several hours of poorly defined abdominal pain. The pain has been intermittent for the previous 3 days and most pronounced postprandial. Her abdominal examination is

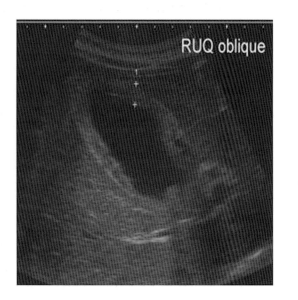

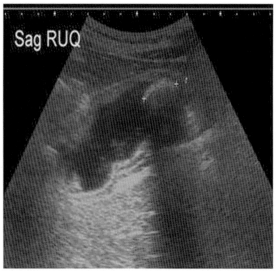

significant for prominent tenderness in both the right upper and lower quadrant. Mild right adnexal tenderness is noted on pelvic examination. The remainder of the examination is unremarkable. A pelvic ultrasound is normal. The patient's abdominal pain progresses while waiting for an abdominal computerized tomography (CT) scan with contrast. Laboratory tests reveal a white blood cell count of 9600/mm³; the serum chemistry, alanine aminotransferase (ALT), aspartate aminotransferase (AST), and serum bilirubin are all normal. A bedside ultrasound of the right upper quadrant is performed, revealing the images noted.

Question: Which of the following statements is most accurate?

A These images reveal a normal gallbladder

B These images reveal gallstones with an otherwise normal gallbladder suggesting the diagnosis of either biliary colic or asymptomatic stones unrelated to the patient's presenting complaint

C These images show no gallstones, but demonstrate evidence of cholecystitis (i.e. acalculous cholecystitis)

D These images reveal gallstones with evidence of cholecystitis

E These images reveal gallstones and an abnormal gallbladder, but decisions regarding cholecystitis need to be made clinically, rendering it unlikely given the patient's history, exam, and laboratory findings

See page 77 for Answer, Diagnosis, and Discussion.

Case 15 | **An elderly man from a house fire**

Christopher P. Holstege, MD

Case presentation: A 74-year-old man presents to the emergency department after being transported by emergency medical services from a house fire. He reportedly had been asleep when the fire broke out. He initially tried to put the fire out, but the fire flashed resulting in extensive burns to his neck, face, arms, and legs. His facial examination is pictured at right. He is complaining of pain at his burn sites and shortness of breath. He is expectorating soot-filled sputum. His vital signs reveal pulse 124, blood pressure 98/54 mmHg, respiratory rate 38 breaths/minute, and temperature 37.1°C. He is orientated to person, place, and time. He has a hoarse voice, audible stridor, diffuse rales on lung examination, and 40% of his body surface area has second and third degree burns.

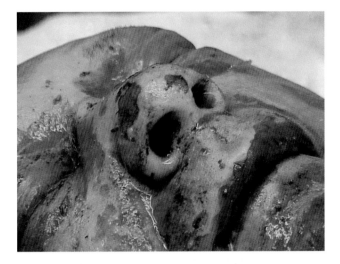

Question: The next correct step in his management includes which of the following?

A Administer intravenous fluids at a maintenance rate of 100 mL/hour

B Administer an intravenous bolus and then maintenance infusion of heparin

C Avoid administration of opioid analgesics to prevent sedation

D Initiate bilevel positive airway pressure (BiPap) to maximize the patient's oxygenation

E Emergent rapid sequence intubation

See page 78 for Answer, Diagnosis, and Discussion.

Case 16 | **Back pain following a fall**

Andrew D. Perron, MD & Christopher T. Bowe, MD

Case presentation: A 78-year-old male patient presents to the emergency department after falling 7 feet from a ladder onto the ground. He noted immediate pain in the lower back. Examination revealed high lumbar tenderness.

Neurologic examination is unremarkable. A radiograph is obtained (see figure).

Question: Which of the following statements is true regarding the management of this patient?
A No further tests are necessary because the patient's neurological exam is normal
B A computerized axial tomography (CT) scan should be performed
C The patient should be placed in a plaster cast and discharged with adequate analgesics
D Ultrasound should be performed of the area to rule-out a significant hematoma
E An epidural nerve block should be performed in the emergency department for pain control

See page 79 for Answer, Diagnosis, and Discussion.

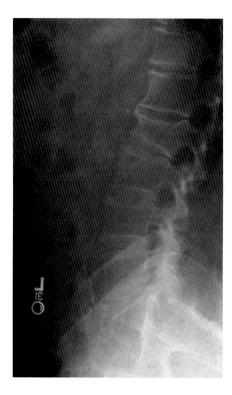

Case 17 | **A bite to the leg in tall grass**

Christopher P. Holstege, MD

Case presentation: A 22-year-old male presents to the emergency department with a complaint that a copperhead had bitten his leg 1 hour ago. He denies any significant pain other than mild discomfort where the fangs broke the skin. He has no nausea or vomiting. The examination of the envenomation site is noted in the figure, with the fang puncture wounds circled. He has no tenderness on palpation of his leg and his leg compartments are soft. He ambulates without difficulty and demonstrates full range of motion of his leg.

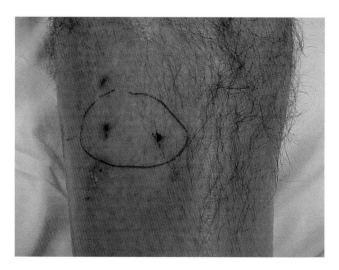

Question: Which of the following would be appropriate in his management?
A Emergent antivenom administration
B Immediate application of a suction devise
C Tourniquet application to his leg
D Discharge to home if no further development of symptoms over the next 4 hours
E Incise the bite site and irrigate the wound

See page 80 for Answer, Diagnosis, and Discussion.

Case 18 | Facial swelling in a patient with poor dentition

Alexander B. Baer, MD & Christopher P. Holstege, MD

Case discussion: A 35-year-old male presents to the emergency department with a complaint of facial discomfort. He developed progressive left molar odontalgia over the preceding week. Over the past 2 days he has been having intermittent fevers and chills. Facial swelling (see figure) began 4 hours prior to arrival. He denies having any dysphagia, dysphonia, or dyspnea.

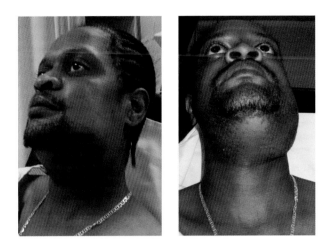

Question: What would be the most appropriate management of this patient?

A Oral penicillin, opioid analgesics, and outpatient follow-up with his dentist

B Subcutaneous epinephrine, intravenous methylprednisolone, and diphenhydramine with admission to a monitored medical floor

C Emergent ultrasound evaluation of the superior vena cava

D Intravenous broad spectrum antibiotics and emergent neck surgery consultation

E Dental alveolar block with lidocaine and outpatient follow-up with dentistry

See page 81 for Answer, Diagnosis, and Discussion.

Case 19 | Elbow pain in a child after a fall

Alexander B. Baer, MD

Case presentation: An 8-year-old child fell from a tree onto his right outstretched arm. He presents to the emergency department 2 hours after the accident with a complaint of elbow pain. The patient describes the pain as a constant ache that is exacerbated with any movement of the arm. On examination, there is moderate swelling localized to the elbow. Elbow pain occurs with passive movement. He has good strength of the hand, and his sensory and vascular exams are normal.

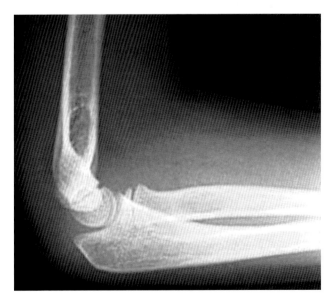

Question: What does this lateral radiograph of the elbow reveal?

A Radial head dislocation

B Capitellum fracture

C Monteggia fracture

D Galeazzi fracture

E Anterior and posterior fat pads

See page 82 for Answer, Diagnosis, and Discussion.

Case 20 | **A man with diffuse facial edema**

Kevin S. Barlotta, MD & Alexander Baer, MD

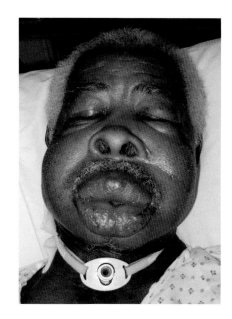

Case presentation: A 63-year-old male with a history of neck cancer and subsequent tracheostomy presents with a complaint of facial "fullness" that rapidly developed over the previous 24 hours. For the past week, he noted mild facial swelling in the morning, but it rapidly resolved as the day progressed. He denies trauma, fever, or dental discomfort. He is taking no new medications and is not on any angiotensin-converting enzyme inhibitors. His facial examination is pictured.

Question: What is the most likely clinical diagnosis?
A Angioedema
B Ludwig's angina
C Bollous pemphigoid
D Superior vena cava syndrome
E Stevens–Johnson syndrome

See page 83 for Answer, Diagnosis, and Discussion.

Case 21 | **Chest pain and hypotension in an adult male patient**

William J. Brady, MD

Case presentation: A 48-year-old man with a history of diabetes mellitus complained of substernal chest pain. On arrival to the emergency department he was pale, diaphoretic, and hypotensive with a blood pressure of 70 mmHg by palpation; the pulmonary examination was unremarkable. An electrocardiogram (ECG) was performed and noted below. Fluid resuscitation was initiated which corrected the hypoperfusion. Laboratory studies and a chest radiograph were obtained while appropriate medications were administered.

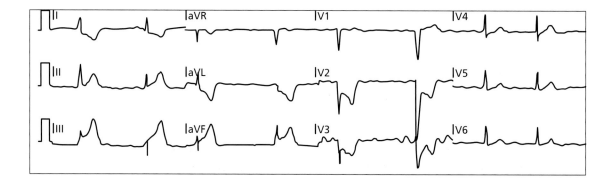

Question: The electrocardiogram reveals:

A Sinus bradycardia with nonspecific ST-segment–T-wave abnormalities

B Sinus bradycardia with inferoposterior RV infarction

C Sinus bradycardia with right ventricular acute myocardial infarction

D Sinus bradycardia with benign early repolarization

E Sinus bradycardia with anterior myocardial infarction

See page 83 for Answer, Diagnosis, and Discussion.

Case 22 | **Eye pain after tree branch strike**

Chris S. Bergstrom, MD & Alexander B. Baer, MD

Case presentation: A 57-year-old patient presents to the emergency department complaining of sharp eye pain, tearing, photophobia, and foreign body sensation after being struck in the left eye with a tree branch.

Physical examination (pictured below left) reveals mildly reduced visual acuity to 20/60 in the left eye. Pupillary examination is normal. The left upper eyelid is slightly edematous and the conjunctiva is injected. The cornea is clear without evidence of an infiltrate. The anterior chamber is deep and clear. The iris and lens are normal.

Instillation of fluorescein reveals an epithelial staining defect with sharp borders measuring 8 mm × 7 mm in size (pictured below right).

Question: Which of the following management plans is the next appropriate step?

A Perform magnetic resonance imaging of the orbit

B Administer adequate analgesics and topical antibiotics

C Perform an emergent lateral canthotomy

D Have the patient insert his contact lens

E Administer oral prednisone

See page 85 for Answer, Diagnosis, and Discussion.

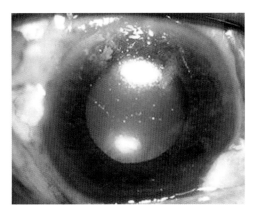
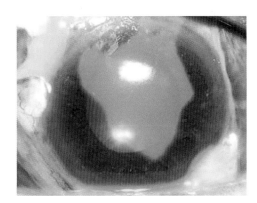

Case 23 | **A missing button battery**

Brendan E. Carr, MD & Sarah G. Winters, MD

Case presentation: A 2-year-old boy presents to the emergency department with a complaint of food intolerance of abrupt onset. His mom reports that he was seen playing with a small calculator just before lunch. She has subsequently noticed that the calculator is missing the back and she is concerned that he has swallowed the battery. On exam, he is in no apparent distress and is tolerating his secretions. His vital signs are normal. An X-ray is obtained (see figure).

Question: What is the next most appropriate management strategy at this time?

A Discharge home and follow with serial outpatient abdominal X-rays

B Administer 25 g of activated charcoal orally

C Admit the patient for intravenous hydration, serial abdominal X-rays, and stool checks to confirm passage

D Infuse 1 mg of glucagon intravenous to decrease lower esophageal sphincter pressure and monitor over the following 6 hours

E Emergent gastroenterology consultation for endoscopic removal of foreign body

See page 85 for Answer, Diagnosis, and Discussion.

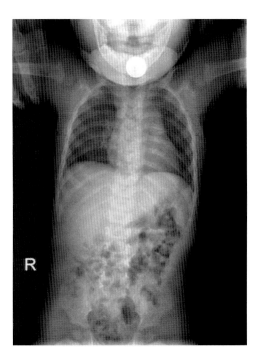

Case 24 | **Acute abdominal pain in pregnancy**

Anthony J. Dean, MD

Case presentation: A 17-year-old female presents to the emergency department with pelvic cramping and vaginal spotting for the past 15 hours. Vital signs are stable. On abdominal exam she has mild lower abdominal tenderness without peritoneal signs. Pelvic exam reveals a closed os and mild bilateral adnexal tenderness. A urine pregnancy test is positive. Blood is obtained for type and screen, and sent for quantitative beta human choriogonadotropin (beta-HCG). A pelvic ultrasound picture is noted below.

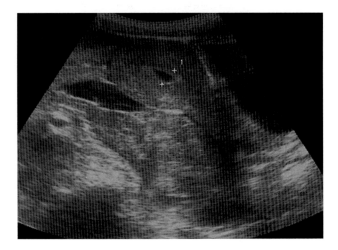

Question: Which of the following is true regarding this midline sagittal transabdominal pelvic sonogram?

A With a quantitative beta-HCG of 452 mIU/mL, the findings of the ultrasound are uninterpretable, since this is below the discriminatory zone.

B This image shows an early gestational sac consistent with a quantitative beta-HCG of 600 mIU/mL. The patient should be told she has an intrauterine pregnancy and should follow-up with her obstetrician for routine prenatal care.

C This image shows an early gestational sac consistent with a quantitative beta-HCG of 321 mIU/mL. The patient should be told she probably has an intrauterine pregnancy. Since this is not definite, it is essential that she follow-up with her obstetrician for a repeat evaluation and quantitative beta-HCG in 2–3 days.

D With a quantitative beta-HCG of 250 mIU/mL, the image shows a probable ectopic pregnancy and the obstetrician should be called for an immediate evaluation in the emergency department.

E With a quantitative beta-HCG of 7430 mIU/mL, this image shows an abnormal intrauterine pregnancy and the patient needs to be referred to obstetrician for evaluation of incomplete abortion.

See page 87 for Answer, Diagnosis, and Discussion.

Case 25 | **Painless penile ulcer**

Andrea L. Neimann, MD

Case presentation: A 35-year-old male presents to the emergency department complaining of a sore that he recently noticed on his penis. He describes the sore as painless and he denies any associated penile discharge. He has never had this problem before. He is currently in a stable relationship with a man and recently had an HIV test which was negative. On exam, there is a single ulcer on the distal end of the penis. The ulcer is 2 cm in diameter and has a slightly raised indurated margin with a clean base. His inguinal lymph nodes are mildly enlarged bilaterally. They feel slightly rubbery, but are discreet and non-tender.

Question: What is the next most appropriate management strategy at this time?

A Discharge the patient to home without treatment

B Treat the patient empirically for herpes

C Be reassured by the patient's reported negative HIV test result and suggest no further testing for HIV in the future

D Treat empirically for syphilis based on the history, physical exam, and knowledge of the epidemiology of genital ulcers in your geographic area

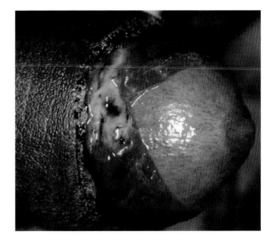

E Perform urinalysis and treat based on the results

See page 88 for Answer, Diagnosis, and Discussion.

Case 26 | **Low back pain in car accident victim**

Edward G. Walsh, MD & William J. Brady, MD

Case presentation: A 48-year-old female was the restrained rear seat passenger in a high-speed motor vehicle crash. The car was traveling approximately 70 miles/hour and hit an oncoming truck that had crossed the median. There was extensive damage to the vehicle and an on-scene fatality was reported by paramedics. During her prolonged extrication the patient complained of immediate lower back pain and lower extremity paresthesia. She was immobilized on-scene and transported to the emergency department. Upon arrival, the patient complained of severe lower back pain and bilateral lower extremity paresthesia. She had a notable "seat-belt sign" across her lower abdomen. Her neurological exam was significant for decreased sensation in both lower extremities and decreased dorsiflexion in both feet. A full trauma evaluation was initiated and multiple radiographs including the one shown were obtained.

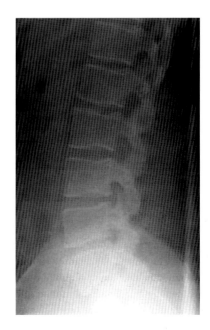

Question: This presentation is consistent with which type of injury?

A T12–L1 dislocation
B L5 teardrop fracture
C L1 transverse process fracture
D L2 pedicle fracture
E L3 burst fracture

See page 89 for Answer, Diagnosis, and Discussion.

Case 27 | **A gardener with a non-healing rash**

Roger A. Band, MD

Case presentation: This 46-year-old gardener presents to a remote clinic in a Guatemalan village. He complains of nodular, erythematous lesions on his right upper extremity. The initial lesion on his distal arm eventually ulcerated and other lesions have been draining non-purulent material. The patient is otherwise without complaints and specifically denies nausea, vomiting, fevers, weight loss, or diarrhea. On exam he appears generally well, with the exception of the impressive lesions seen in the pictures on his right upper extremity.

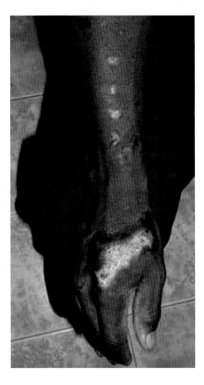

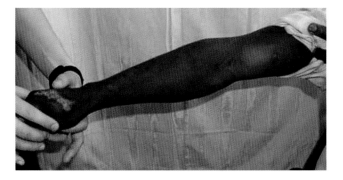

Question: What is the most likely cause for these lesions?

A Methicillin-resistant *Staphylococcus aureus*
B Scalding injury
C Scabies
D Sporotrichosis
E Tuberculosis

See page 90 for Answer, Diagnosis, and Discussion.

Case 28 | **An immigrant with neck swelling**

Suzanne M. Shepherd, MD, Anthony J. Dean, MD & William H. Shoff, MD

Case presentation: A 45-year-old male immigrant from Morocco presents with neck discomfort and swelling. Three months prior the area was initially swollen with only a single mass noted. Over the last month, the area began to drain and he has noted an increase in the number of masses. He also has had an unexpected 30-pound weight loss over the last year with associated night sweats. He denies other illnesses. He lives alone and is employed as a taxi driver.

His examination is unremarkable except for the neck exam depicted in the picture. There are also multiple 2–6 cm, matted, soft, and – in one case – fluctuant, mildly tender masses along the posterior cervical chain.

Question: Which of the following illnesses would be the most likely cause of this patient's illness?
A Mononucleosis
B Streptococcal pharyngitis
C Cytomegalovirus
D Tuberculosis
E Toxoplasmosis

See page 90 for Answer, Diagnosis, and Discussion.

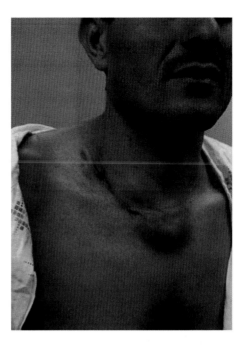

Case 29 | **Fall on an outstretched hand in a young adolescent**

William J. Brady, MD & Kevin S. Barlotta, MD

Case presentation: A 13-year-old male was playing soccer when, at full sprint, he tripped and fell. Both upper extremities were extended fully when he impacted the ground on his outstretched hands. Immediately upon falling, he noted pain in

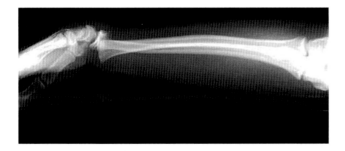

the right wrist. On examination, he had tenderness in the region of the distal radius with overlying soft tissue swelling. Radiographs were performed and one is noted here.

Question: The patient can expect the following outcome from this injury assuming adequate care is provided:
A Complete growth arrest at this injury site with arm length shortening
B Complete recovery with normal growth
C Chronic pain with osteo-necrosis at the injury site
D Chronic disability as a consequence of this injury
E High risk for the development of compartment syndrome

See page 91 for Answer, Diagnosis, and Discussion.

Case 30 | **Raccoon eyes**

Angela M. Mills, MD

Case presentation: A 25-year-old male was involved in a motorcycle crash without a helmet. The patient had a

documented loss of consciousness at the scene and presents with a complaint of head pain, dizziness, and nausea. On exam there is mild confusion, the findings as shown in the figure, and a non-focal neurological exam.

Question: What is the next most appropriate management strategy at this time?

A Recommend analgesics, ice, and follow-up care
B Emergent lateral canthotomy
C Order a skull radiograph
D Order a head computed axial tomography (CT) scan for possible intracranial injury
E Administer mannitol and dexamethasone emergently

See page 92 for Answer, Diagnosis, and Discussion.

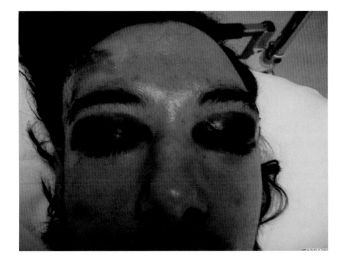

Case 31 | **Chest pain and a confounding electrocardiogram pattern**

William J. Brady, MD

Case presentation: A 67-year-old male with a past history of coronary artery disease, diabetes mellitus, and hypertension presented to the emergency department with substernal chest pain. The pain had appeared approximately 2 hours ago and was associated with diaphoresis and nausea. The patient was treated for acute cardiac ischemia. A 12-lead electrocardiogram (ECG) is performed and noted below.

Question: Which of the following is the correct statement regarding the ECG presentation of left bundle branch block (LBBB) and possible acute myocardial infarction (AMI)?

A LBBB pattern does not confound the clinician's ability to use the ECG to diagnose AMI

B Discordant ST segments are most often normal in the LBBB pattern
C Concordant ST segment elevation is a normal finding in the LBBB pattern
D LBBB pattern is not associated with an increased risk of poor outcome in acute coronary syndrome (ACS) patients
E The longer the QRS duration, the greater the risk for ACS

See page 93 for Answer, Diagnosis, and Discussion.

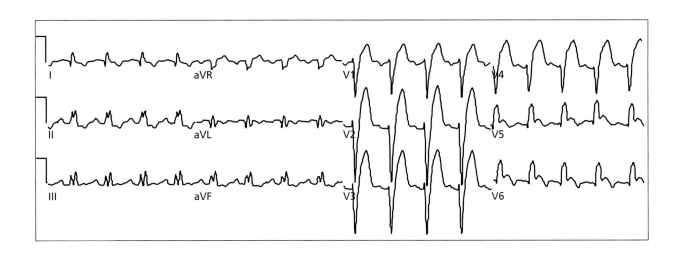

Case 32 | **Eye pain in a contact lens wearer**

Chris S. Bergstrom, MD & Alexander B. Baer, MD

Case presentation: A 27-year-old soft contact lens wearer presents with a complaint of redness, blurred vision, pain, and photophobia in the right eye. The patient admits to "over wearing" her contact lenses, and sleeps in them on a regular basis. She also states that her eyes are matted together in the morning.

On physical examination, the visual acuity is reduced to 20/100 in the right eye. The pupil examination is normal. The conjunctiva is injected and there is a 4 mm oval, white, fluffy opacity on the cornea as noted in the figure.

Slit lamp examination reveals cell and flare in the anterior chamber. The iris and lens detail are obscured by the opacity but are otherwise normal.

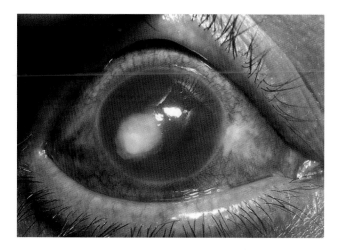

Question: What is the appropriate management for this condition?
A Topical steroid
B Topical antiviral agent
C Topical antibiotics
D Burr removal of this foreign body
E Oral antiviral agent

See page 94 for Answer, Diagnosis, and Discussion.

Case 33 | **Heel pain following a fall**

David F. Gaieski, MD

Case presentation: A 26-year-old roofer fell off a 12-foot-high roof and landed on the pavement below. He was wearing steel-toed construction boots and landed directly on his left heel in a standing position. He felt extreme pain in his heel after the fall and was unable to ambulate at the scene. His co-workers called emergency medical services and he was placed in spinal immobilization and transported to the emergency department. On arrival, he complained of left heel pain and midline low back pain. His examination revealed a markedly swollen heel with ecchymosis and tenderness to palpation over the plantar surface of his hind-foot. Examination of his back revealed bilateral paraspinous muscle tenderness to palpation without midline bony tenderness. An intravenous line was placed, he was given morphine for pain control, and a foot radiograph series was significant for the finding pictured.

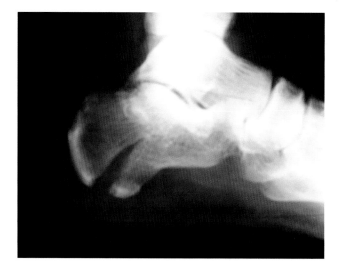

Question: The next most appropriate step in the management of this man's injury is:

A Plaster cast immobilization, pain control, and orthopedic outpatient follow-up

B Radiographs of the lumbar spine to rule out accompanying fracture; orthopedic consultation for possible operative intervention

C Crutches, non-weight-bearing, pain control, follow-up with his family physician

D Posterior splint, non-weight-bearing, pain control, orthopedic follow-up for rigid cast in 3–5 days

E Fracture closed reduction and posterior splint

See page 94 for Answer, Diagnosis, and Discussion.

Case 34 | FAST evaluation following trauma

Bon S. Ku, MD & Anthony J. Dean, MD

Case presentation: A 25-year-old unrestrained driver presents to the emergency department after a motor vehicle crash. En route to the hospital he receives 1 L of intravenous lactated ringers. He arrives with the following vital signs: blood pressure 90/70 mmHg, pulse 120 beats/minute, respirations 22 breaths/minute, oxygen saturation of 100%. He has a Glasgow coma scale of 15, facial contusions and lacerations, with "tingling" in his hands bilaterally. He complains of pain "everywhere." Neurological exam reveals decreased sensation in both hands. A focused assessment by sonography in trauma (FAST) is performed and is noted right.

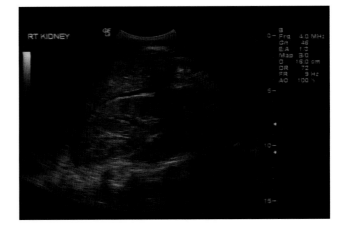

Question: Which of the following describes the patient's condition and the next most appropriate action in his management?

A The ultrasound shows no significant abnormality. If the rest of the FAST is negative, the patient should be transfused with whole blood, and once stabilized, cervical cord trauma is his most urgent issue. His neck should be immobilized and evaluated by a neurosurgeon.

B The ultrasound image suggests <200 mL of free fluid. The patient should be transfused with whole blood, sent to computerized tomography (CT) for evaluation of the abdomen, and observed with serial abdominal exams.

C The ultrasound image suggests >200 mL of free fluid. The patient should be transfused with whole blood, sent to CT for evaluation of the abdomen, and observed with serial abdominal exams.

D The ultrasound suggests <200 mL of free fluid. The patient should have immediate surgical evaluation in preparation for transfer to the operating room for exploratory laparotomy.

E The ultrasound suggests >200 mL of free fluid. The patient should have immediate surgical evaluation in preparation for transfer to the operating room for exploratory laparotomy.

See page 95 for Answer, Diagnosis, and Discussion.

Case 35 | Skin lesion in a heroin addict

Christopher P. Holstege, MD & Alexander B. Baer, MD

Case presentation: A 42-year-old female with a history of hepatitis C presents to the emergency department with a complaint of left hand pain that she attributes to a "chronic skin condition." Examination of her hand is significant for the findings shown in the figure. Peripheral intravenous access was attempted without success. The patient was discovered to have extensive scarring along her bilateral femoral and external jugular veins.

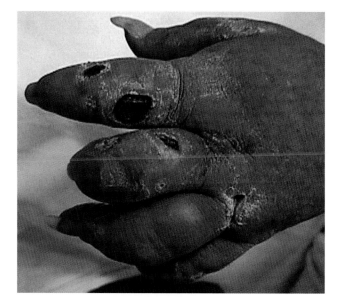

Question: Which of the following best describes her skin condition?
A Grand central station
B Skin popping
C Acne vulgaris
D Pocketing
E Acne cystica

See page 96 for Answers, Diagnosis, and Discussion.

Case 36 | **Young athlete with back pain**

Edward G. Walsh, MD & William J. Brady, MD

Case presentation: A 20-year-old man returns to the emergency department with a chief complaint of lower back pain. He has been seen twice previously for the same complaint. There is no history of trauma or overuse. He plays tennis regularly and runs 3–5 miles nearly every day of the week. He has been unable to exercise regularly since his symptoms began 3 months ago. He has noted some bilateral hamstring tightness but no other symptoms or neurological deficits. His physical exam is benign except for tenderness and mild bilateral paraspinous muscle spasm over L5. His pain noticeably worsened on extension of his lower spine. Radiographs were obtained (see figure).

Question: This clinical presentation is most consistent with:
A L5 discitis
B Juvenile rheumatoid arthritis
C Sciatica
D L5 pars defect
E Transverse myelitis

See page 98 for Answer, Diagnosis, and Discussion.

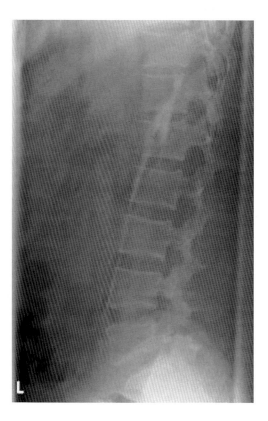

Case 37 | Skin lesions in a comatose patient

Christopher P. Holstege, MD

Case presentation: A 24-year-old male presents to the emergency department following an overdose of multiple pills, including sedatives. He was intubated on the scene by

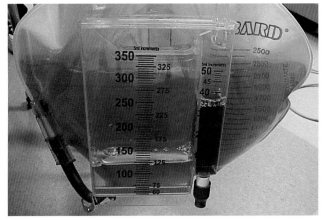

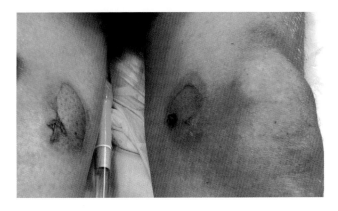

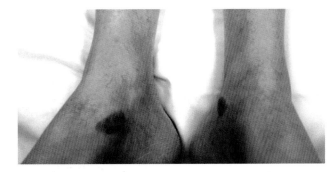

paramedics and transported to the hospital. On examination of the patient, the skin lesions pictured left are discovered.

A Foley catheter is placed with return of the urine pictured above.

Question: Which of the following is the most appropriate initial therapy?
A Apply silver sulfadiazine cream to the wounds
B Administer intravenous broad spectrum antibiotics
C Administer adequate intravenous fluids to assure an adequate urine output
D Perform emergent fasciotomy in the emergency department
E Administer intravenous potassium

See page 99 for Answer, Diagnosis, and Discussion.

Case 38 | Chest pain with sudden cardiac death

William J. Brady, MD

Case presentation: A 65-year-old man presented to the emergency department with chest pain and syncope. The examination demonstrated an alert man in mild distress with normal vital signs; diaphoresis was present on the examination. The patient suddenly slumped over; he was

unresponsive without pulse. The cardiac rhythm strip below was obtained.

While attempts were made for electrical therapy, the rhythm changed spontaneously to sinus rhythm with a pulse. A 12-lead electrocardiogram was obtained and is

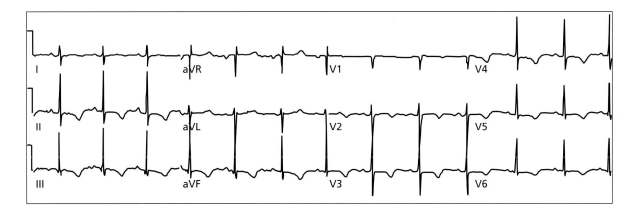

noted above. Additional diagnostic studies were performed while therapy was initiated.

Question: Which of the following would be consistent with the rhythm strip and electrocardiogram noted in this case?
A Hypercalcemia
B Hyperchloremia
C Hypernatremia
D Hypomagnesemia
E Hypophosphatemia

See page 100 for Answer, Diagnosis, and Discussion.

Case 39 | **Fall on an outstretched hand with wrist pain**

William J. Brady, MD & Kevin S. Barlotta, MD

Case presentation: A 28-year-old male patient presents to the emergency department after sustaining a fall on his out-stretched hand (FOOSH). He noted immediate pain but denied other complaints. Examination revealed snuffbox tenderness. The radiograph as shown was obtained.

Question: In the patient with a FOOSH mechanism with palpable snuffbox tenderness and a non-diagnostic radiograph, which management course should be pursued?
A Discharge home with non-steroidal anti-inflammatory therapy and no scheduled outpatient physician follow-up.
B Discharge home, prescribe appropriate analgesic therapy, and splint the wrist with instructions to leave in place for 1 week at which time the patient can resume normal activity.
C Inform the patient that he may have an occult wrist fracture, splint the wrist, prescribe appropriate analgesic therapy, and arrange close physician outpatient follow-up.
D Perform magnetic resonance imaging (MRI) at initial evaluation with emergent orthopedic surgery consultation.
E Perform fracture reduction under conscious sedation and cast the wrist.

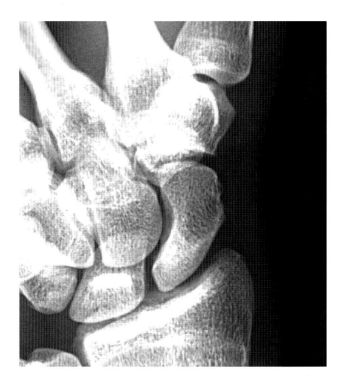

See page 101 for Answer, Diagnosis, and Discussion.

Case 40 | **Necrotic skin lesion**

David A. Kasper, MBA, Aradhna Saxena, MD & Kenneth A. Katz, MD

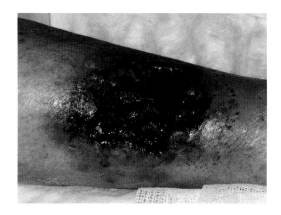

Case presentation: A 57-year-old Caucasian man complains of an expanding "spider bite" on his left pretibial area. He noticed the lesion 3 days prior as a painful and progressively enlarging "pimple." His medical history is notable for ulcerative colitis, which is currently being treated with mesalamine. On exam, an ulcer with a partially rolled, violaceous border and a black eschar is present on the left pretibial area. There is no lower extremity edema. The patient is otherwise well.

Question: What is the next most appropriate management strategy at this time?

A Empirical treatment with broad-spectrum antibiotics
B Debridement of the eschar
C Consult dermatology for biopsy of ulcer for tissue culture and histology

D Treatment with compression stockings
E Brown Recluse antivenom infusion

See page 102 for Answer, Diagnosis, and Discussion.

Case 41 | **Chest pain with electrocardiographic ST-segment/T-wave abnormalities**

William J. Brady, MD

Case presentation: A 55-year-old female with a history of hypertension presented to the emergency department with chest pain. The physical examination was unremarkable. The initial 12-lead electrocardiogram (ECG) is noted

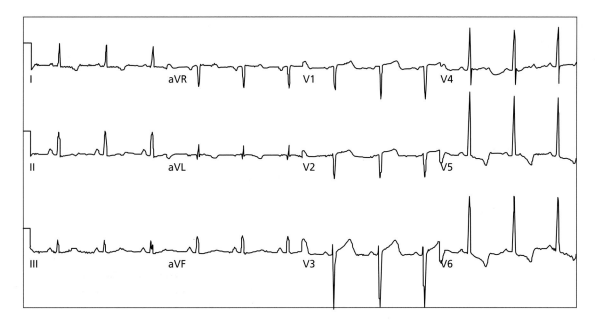

here. The patient received nitroglycerin and aspirin with resolution of the pain. Serial ECGs did not reveal interval change; laboratory studies were negative. The patient ruled out for myocardial infarction.

Question: ECG left ventricular hypertrophy:

A Confounds the ECG diagnosis of acute myocardial infarction

B Does not reduce the ECG's ability to diagnose acute coronary syndrome

C Is always associated with ST-segment/T-wave changes

D Is an indication for fibrinolysis

E Is always associated with hypertension

See page 103 for Answer, Diagnosis, and Discussion.

Case 42 | **Chemical eye exposure**

Chris S. Bergstrom, MD & Alexander B. Baer, MD

Case presentation: A 34-year-old female is seen in the emergency department after having an unknown chemical splashed in her face and eyes. She is complaining of burning, tearing, decreased vision, and light sensitivity. Gross inspection reveals first degree burns to the periorbital skin and lids. The globes are intact.

On physical examination (see figure) the visual acuity is 20/200 in each eye. The bulbar and palpebral conjunctiva is markedly injected with a watery mucous discharge. The corneas are hazy with blurred iris detail. There is a 6 mm oval area of blanched bulbar conjunctiva inferiorly near the limbus. The anterior chambers are deep and the pupils are round.

Question: What emergent action should be initiated prior to completing the ophthalmic examination?

A Emergent ophthalmology consultation

B Litmus test

C Irrigation of the eye with copious fluids such as saline or lactated ringers

D Tetanus prophylaxis

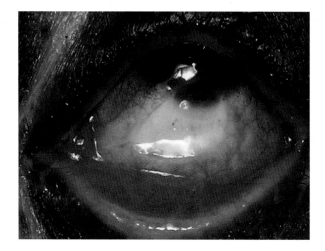

E Neutralization with a weak acid or base for a base- or acid-offending agent, respectively

See page 104 for Answer, Diagnosis, and Discussion.

Case 43 | **Hand pain after striking a wall**

William J. Brady, MD & Kevin S. Barlotta, MD

Case presentation: A 24-year-old intoxicated male presents to the emergency department after striking a wall at an oblique angle. He noted significant pain in his hand and denied any other complaints. On examination, the hand demonstrated significant tenderness and soft tissue swelling in the medial-dorsal area. Radiographs, an anteroposterior view of the hand/wrist and lateral view of the hand/wrist, were obtained as shown in the figures.

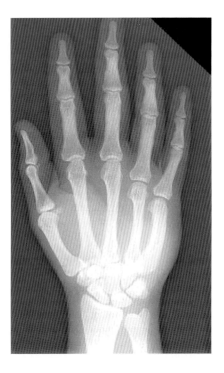

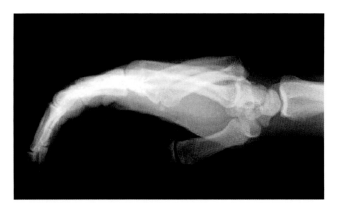

Question: The most likely injury in this type of presentation is:

A Closed fist injury with a "fight bite"
B Scaphoid fracture
C Carpometacarpal dislocation
D Scapholunate dissociation
E Radial head fracture

See page 104 for Answer, Diagnosis, and Discussion.

Case 44 | **Dyspnea in an alcoholic**

Anthony J. Dean, MD

Case presentation: A 50-year-old alcohol abuser presents complaining of shortness of breath and abdominal and back pain "like my pancreas". The patient is agitated and refuses to lie down. She is a heavy smoker and noncompliant with medications for hypertension. The patient denies trauma but has contusions and abrasions on her hands and arms in various stages of healing. Her vitals are blood pressure 106/85 mmHg, heart rate 124 beats/minute, respiratory rate 32/minute. Pulse oximetry is 90% on 2 L nasal cannula. With examination limited by the patient's inability to cooperate, the following are noted: dry mucous membranes, no jugular venous distension, distant heart sounds, and grossly symmetric breath sounds. The following bedside ultrasound images are obtained by the examining physician.

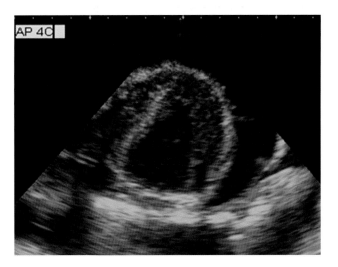

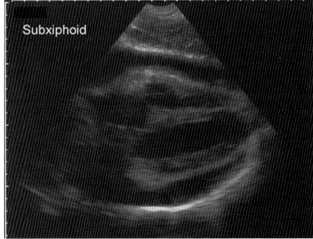

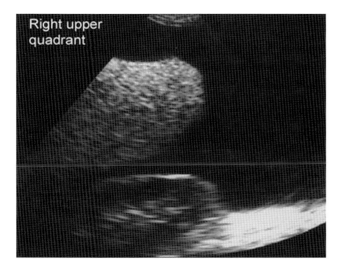

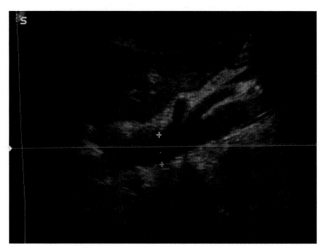

Question: Which of the following is true?

A With these images, the patient should be sent for emergent head computerized tomography (CT) to exclude intracranial vascular catastrophe as a cause for her abnormal mental status.

B These images demonstrate intraperitoneal fluid suggestive of hemorrhage. Whether this is due to acute aortic aneurysm or occult trauma, the patient requires immediate surgical evaluation for possible emergent operative management.

C These images, combined with the absence of muffled heart sounds, jugular venous distension,

and hypotension, make tamponade exceedingly unlikely.

D These images show pericardial effusion with evidence of dissection in the abdominal aorta. This suggests an acute proximal dissection, mandating immediate consultation with a cardiothoracic surgeon for operative repair.

E These images show large pericardial effusion. The diagnosis of tamponade will be made based on a dynamic assessment of cardiac filling during diastole.

See page 105 for Answer, Diagnosis, and Discussion.

Case 45 | **Slash wound to the neck**

Kevin S. Barlotta, MD & Alexander B. Baer, MD

Case presentation: A 35-year-old female presents to the emergency department after an altercation. She states that she was attacked with a hunting knife. She complains of

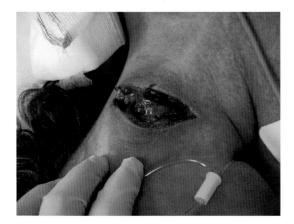

only pain at the wound site. She denies voice changes or difficulty swallowing. Her injury is depicted left.

Question: What zone of injury is represented in the image?

A Zone I

B Zone II

C Zone III

D Zone IV

E Zone 0

See page 107 for Answer, Diagnosis, and Discussion.

Case 46 | Foot pain following breaking

Munish Goyal, MD

Case presentation: A 22-year-old female presents to the emergency department with left foot pain. She was the

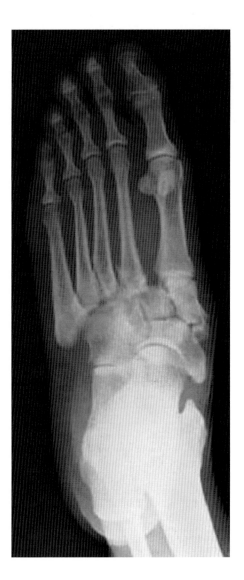

restrained driver of a car which struck another car head-on. She used her left foot to compress the brake pedal just prior to impact. She complains of decreased movement of her toes and says she can't walk on her left foot. She denies loss of consciousness or any other complaints. Her foot appears mildly swollen, is exquisitely tender along the midfoot, and has normal distal pulses and capillary refill. The following foot radiographs obtained are ordered from triage.

Question: What is the most appropriate management strategy at this time?
A Place the patient in a posterior splint, give her crutches, and refer her to an orthopedic specialist as an outpatient
B Obtain an orthopedic consult, send pre-operative labs, and offer the patient analgesics
C Obtain an emergent angiogram to rule out a vascular injury
D Obtain an emergent orthopedic consult, administer conscious sedation, and perform an emergent reduction
E Administer a hematoma block and perform an emergent reduction

See page 108 for Answer, Diagnosis, and Discussion.

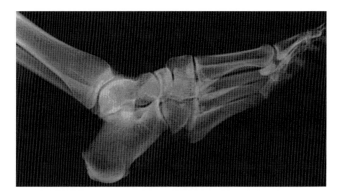

Case 47 | Confluent rash in a child

Sarah G. Winters, MD & Brendan E. Carr, MD

Case presentation: A 2-year-old boy with no medical history presents to the emergency department with complaints

of a diffuse rash over bilateral lower extremities for the past 2 days that is now progressing to his trunk and upper

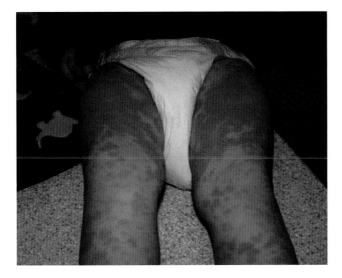

detergents, creams, or drug exposures. His parents report mild upper respiratory symptoms 1 week ago. On physical exam he has multiple confluent lesions with central clearing diffusely. The lesions are present on palms and soles but are most prominent on his bilateral lower extremities. There is no conjunctival injection and there are no sores in or around his mouth or genital area.

Question: What is the next most appropriate management strategy at this time?

A Obtain complete blood count (CBC) and blood culture, administer ceftriaxone, and admit for observation

B Obtain CBC and blood culture, but do not treat with antibiotics

C Discharge to home with diphenlhydramine as needed for itching

D Consult dermatology emergently

E Administer subcutaneous epinephrine immediately

extremities. He is otherwise playful and well appearing with no complaint of itching or fever. His parents deny new

See page 109 for Answer, Diagnosis, and Discussion.

Case 48 | **Lost in the cold**

Adam K. Rowden, DO & Christopher P. Holstege, MD

Case presentation: A 38-year-old male presents to the emergency department after being lost in the wilderness. His feet and legs (pictured in the figure) are ice cold with poor pulses. He complains of marked pain and numbness of his lower extremities. His vital signs are normal, including a core body temperature of 37.1°C.

Question: Which of the following is the most appropriate initial management?

A Gradual rewarming with infrared warming lights

B Rapid rewarming of the afflicted extremities in a warm water (40–42°C) bath for 30 minutes

C Urgent surgical consultation for early debridement and fasciotomy

D Vigorous massage in addition to rewarming

E Heparin therapy and administration of warm intravenous fluids

See page 109 for Answer, Diagnosis, and Discussion.

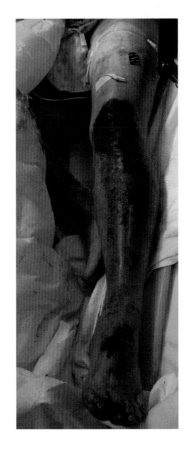

Case 49 | **Bradycardia following an herbal ingestion**

Alexander B. Baer, MD

Case presentation: A 23-year-old male native of Hong Kong presents with near syncope after a prodrome that included nausea, vomiting, extremity paresthesias, and dyspnea. The initial vital signs are pulse 32 beats/minute, blood pressure 75/32 mmHg, respirations 22 breaths/minute. The remainder of his physical examination is unremarkable. The family brings in an herbal product with a picture of this plant on the label.

Question: What would be the next most appropriate step in his management?
A Administer intravenous epinephrine
B Administer intravenous physostigmine
C Administer intravenous adenosine
D Administer intravenous diltiazem
E Administer intravenous atropine

See page 110 for Answer, Diagnosis, and Discussion.

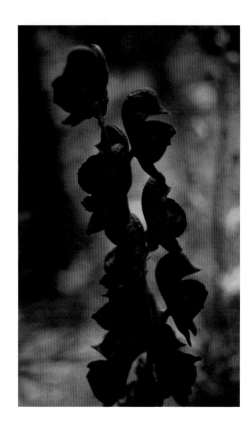

Case 50 | **Abdominal pain in an alcoholic**

Angela M. Mills, MD

Case presentation: A 45-year-old male with a history of alcohol abuse presents to the emergency department with midepigastric abdominal pain radiating straight through to his back and associated with nausea and vomiting. His laboratory values are consistent with the diagnosis of acute pancreatitis. A plain film of the abdomen is obtained.

Question: What is the name of this radiologic finding?
A Double bubble sign
B Target sign
C Sentinel loop
D String of pearls sign
E Coffee-bean sign

See page 111 for Answer, Diagnosis, and Discussion.

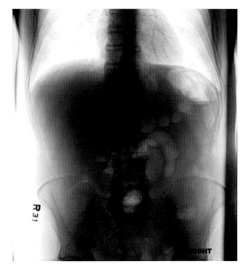

Case 51 | **Pain out of proportion to examination**

Adam K. Rowden, DO

Case presentation: A 47-year-old female presents with severe leg pain and swelling over the past 12 hours. She was working in her yard 2 days ago and sustained a small puncture wound to the area. She describes the initial wound as trivial. One day following the original injury, the pain began and steadily increased; she now cannot bear weight or ambulate. She has had low-grade fevers at home along with generalized malaise. Her vitals are significant for pulse 125 beats/minute, a blood pressure 88/43 mmHg, respirations 28/minute, temperature 38.1°C. Physical examination of her leg is pictured below. Her exam is hampered due to the extreme pain induced with even light touch and passive motion her leg.

An X-ray is obtained and is noted below.

Question: Which of the following is most appropriate in the management of this patient's wound?

A Thorough wound irrigation, tetanus prophylaxis, pain control, oral antibiotics, and outpatient follow-up in 1 week.

B Pain control, tetanus prophylaxis, one dose of intravenous antibiotics in the emergency department and outpatient follow-up in 48 hours.

C Tetanus prophylaxis and pain control. Follow-up outpatient in 5 days.

D Tetanus prophylaxis, thorough wound irrigation, pain control, and inpatient admission to general medicine for intravenous antibiotics.

E Intravenous antibiotics, fluid resuscitation, and emergent surgical consultation for wound debridement.

See page 111 for Answer, Diagnosis, and Discussion.

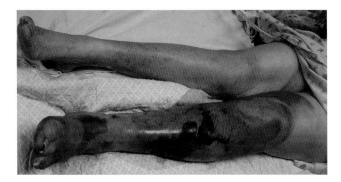 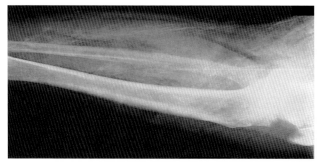

Case 52 | **Pleuritic chest pain in a young adult male**

William J. Brady, MD

Case presentation: A 32-year-old male without medical history presented via ambulance to the emergency department with chest pain. The pain was left-sided in location and worsened upon both inspiration and reclining. The examination revealed a young patient in moderate distress due to chest pain. A rhythm strip and a 12-lead electrocardiogram (ECG) were noted (see figures). Laboratory studies were normal and a chest radiograph revealed a normal heart size and lung fields. The patient received intravenous morphine sulfate and ketorolac, which reduced the pain.

Question: The ECG in a patient with the disease represented in this case can show all of the following except:

A Diffuse ST segment elevation

B Electrical alternans

C PR segment changes

D Prominent Q waves

E T-wave inversion

See page 112 for Answer, Diagnosis, and Discussion.

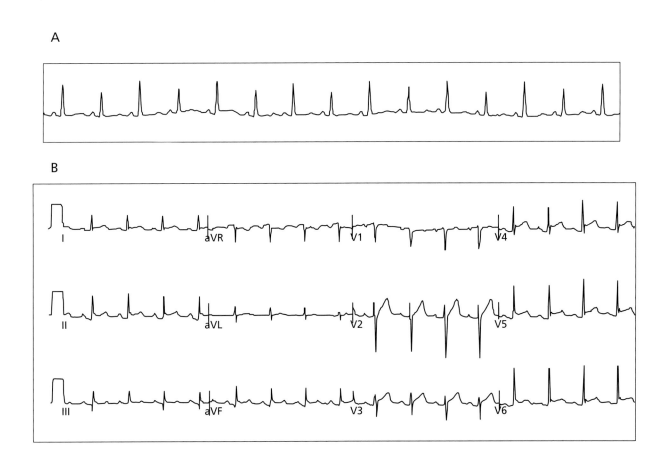

A

B

Case 53 | **Eye pain following a bar fight**

Chris S. Bergstrom, MD & Alexander B. Baer, MD

Case presentation: A 35-year-old male is seen in the emergency department after a bar fight. He has several facial lacerations from a broken bottle. He is complaining of mild periorbital pain and epiphora. On physical examination his visual acuity is 20/30 in the left eye. His pupils are equally round and responsive to direct and consensual stimulation. There is a superficial laceration of the upper lid that does not involve the lid margin and without evidence of prolapsed orbital fat. The lower lid has two full thickness lacerations through the lid margin, one of which is medial to the lower punctum. The conjunctiva, sclera, and cornea are normal. The anterior chamber is deep and clear. The iris is normal and the pupil is round.

Question: Periorbital laceration with prolapsed orbital fat implies damage to what structure?

A Optic nerve
B Lacrimal drainage system
C Cornea
D Orbital septum
E Anterior maxillary wall

See page 112 for Answer, Diagnosis, and Discussion.

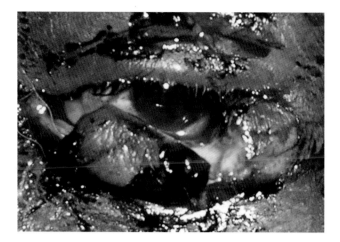

Case 54 | **Forearm fracture after falling**

Alexander B. Baer, MD

Case presentation: A 20-year-old male fell on an outstretched upper extremity while snowboarding. He presents with obvious arm deformity. Radiographs of the elbow are obtained and are pictured below.

Question: What is the name of the fracture pictured in the radiographs?

A Boxer's fracture
B Tear drop fracture
C Tillaux fracture
D Galeazzi fracture
E Monteggia fracture

See page 113 for Answer, Diagnosis, and Discussion.

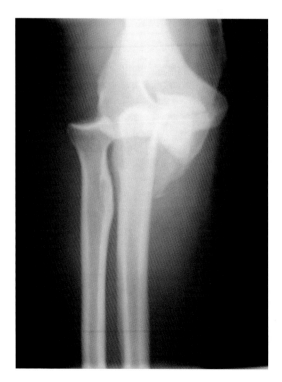

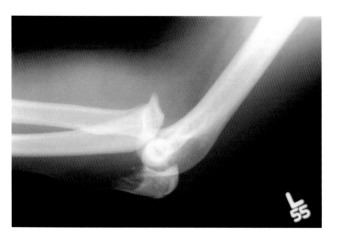

Case 55 | **An elderly woman with groin pain**

Brendan E. Carr, MD

Case presentation: A 65-year-old woman presents to the emergency department with the complaint of atraumatic progressive groin and buttock pain over the last several months. She has curtailed her activities and is now unable to ambulate. Her past medical history is significant only for sarcoidosis and end stage renal disease. She is currently taking prednisone. On exam, there is pain with range of motion and axial load of the left hip. The X-ray shown right is obtained.

Question: All of the following are associated with this condition EXCEPT:
A Corticosteroids
B Sarcoidosis
C Sickle cell disease
D Previous hip fracture or dislocation
E Renal disease

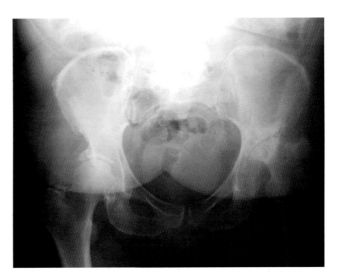

See page 114 for Answer, Diagnosis, and Discussion.

Case 56 | **Painful facial rash**

Chris S. Bergstrom, MD & Alexander B. Baer, MD

Case presentation: A 63-year-old male is seen in the emergency department complaining of a painful rash over the left side of his forehead along with blurred vision, redness, and light sensitivity in the left eye. He states that his symptoms started yesterday. Ocular examination reveals a vesicular rash on the left side of the forehead that respects the midline and involves the upper lid but does not affect the tip of the nose. There is a mucous discharge present. Slit lamp examination shows conjunctival injection. The cornea is clear without evidence of staining or infiltrates. The anterior chamber is deep and quiet. The iris and lens are normal.

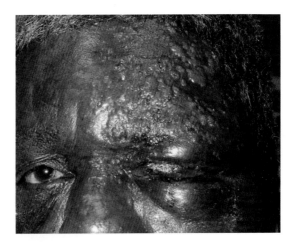

Question: What is Hutchinson's sign?
A Scrapings of the rash demonstrate hyphae when exposed to potassium hydroxide
B Rash involvement of the tympanic membrane
C Fluorescence of the rash when placed under a Wood's lamp
D Rash involvement of the cornea
E Rash involvement of the nose

See page 114 for Answer, Diagnosis, and Discussion.

Case 57 | Confusion, anemia, and abdominal pain in a toddler

Alexander B. Baer, MD & Christopher P. Holstege, MD

Case presentation: A 4-year-old child was seen 3 weeks ago by his pediatrician for abdominal cramping and constipation. The child is an immigrant from Africa and has no significant past medical history. The laboratory evaluation performed during the last office visit demonstrated a hypochromic, microcytic anemia which was thought to be secondary to iron deficiency. The child now presents to the emergency department with anorexia, increasing lethargy, and ataxia. The radiograph shown right is obtained.

Question: What is the treatment of choice for this child?
A D-penicillamine
B 2,3-dimercaptosuccinic acid (DMSA or succimer)
C Calcium disodium ethylene diamine tetraacetate (CaNa2EDTA)
D Dimercaprol (British Antilewisite or BAL)
E Deferoxamine

See page 115 for Answer, Diagnosis, and Discussion.

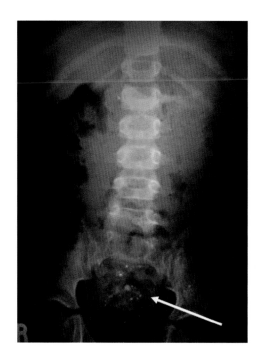

Case 58 | Cardiotoxic effects following caustic ingestion

Alexander B. Baer, MD & Christopher P. Holstege, MD

Case presentation: A previously healthy 47-year-old male accidentally ingested a blue liquid he thought was a sport drink. He immediately noted throat irritation and within 5 minutes of the ingestion, he developed nausea and vomiting. He presented to the emergency department within 1 hour of the ingestion with a complaint of nausea, weakness, and intense pleuritic chest pain. His initial vital signs revealed temperature 34.5°C, pulse 130 beats/minute, blood pressure 102/66 mmHg, and respirations 20 breaths/minute. His voice was hoarse and he had difficulty swallowing his secretions. His exam was significant for an oropharynx with inflamed mucosa and an abdomen that was soft with mild tenderness diffusely.

His initial electrocardiogram (ECG 1, see figure on next page) 1 hour after ingestion was pictured on the next page. His initial arterial blood gas revealed pH 7.28, pCO$_2$ 29, pO$_2$ of 209, and HCO$_3$ 13. Within one and half hour of his arrival, he became increasingly agitated and his systolic blood pressure dropped to 80 mmHg. A repeat ECG (ECG 2) was noted (see figure on next page). Initial bedside evaluation of the ingested fluid by litmus paper revealed a pH less than 4.0.

Question: What electrolyte abnormality is most likely present on laboratory analysis?
A Hypermagnesemia
B Hypocalcemia
C Hypochloremia
D Hypernatremia
E Hypophosphatemia

See page 115 for Answer, Diagnosis, and Discussion.

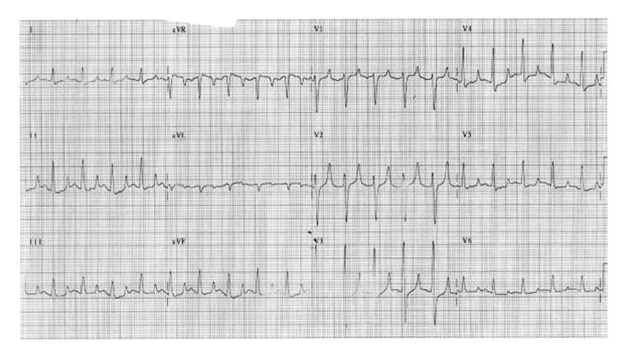

ECG 1.

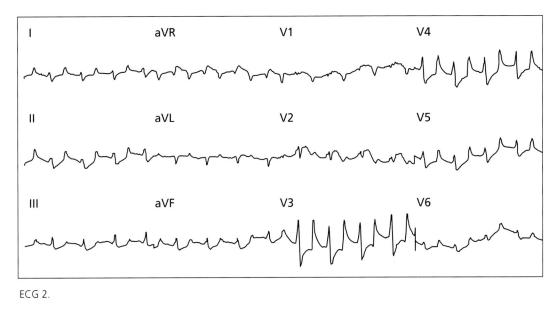

ECG 2.

Case 59 | **Rash and joint pain in a child**

Mara Becker, MD

Case presentation: An 8-year-old boy presents to the emergency department with a rash for 2 days and an inability to ambulate due to bilateral ankle pain. The family reports that the rash began on his legs and is now more generalized. It is not painful nor pruritic. The child is well appearing with normal vital signs. The skin lesions (see figures on the next page) are palpable and purple in hue and do not blanch with pressure. The ankles are warm to the touch and have minimal periarticular swelling, but no intra-articular fluid. On exam the right wrist is also painful and warm with periarticular swelling. The rest of the exam is normal. Laboratory tests reveal a normal complete blood count, coagulation studies, electrolytes, and urinalysis. A blood culture is pending.

Question: What would be the next step in managing this patient?

A Discharge home with close follow-up by the primary care doctor and anti-inflammatory medications for the joint pain

B Admit for observation

C Admit for intravenous antibiotic therapy

D Consult orthopedics for an ankle arthrocentesis

E Administer subcutaneous epinephrine

See page 116 for Answer, Diagnosis, and Discussion.

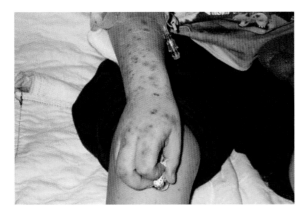

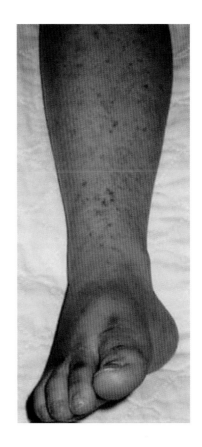

Case 60 | X-ray findings after laparoscopy

Munish Goyal, MD

Case presentation: A 65-year-old male presents to the emergency department with mild abdominal pain. He is 2 days post-laparoscopic cholecystectomy and notes pain at one of his incision sites, worse when he ambulates. He is tolerating a normal diet without nausea or vomiting, had a normal bowel movement today, and is urinating without difficulty. His abdominal incisions are well healing without erythema, fluctuance, or drainage. His abdomen is soft, with mild incision tenderness, normal bowel sounds, and without distension. The plain film (see figure) is ordered from triage.

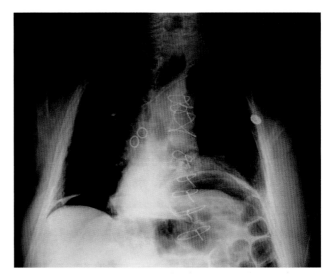

Question: The X-ray findings are consistent with which of the following?

A Pneumonia

B Post-operative pneumoperitoneum

C Large bowel obstruction

D Biliary air

E Kidney stone

See page 117 for Answer, Diagnosis, and Discussion.

Case 61 | Injector injury to the hand

Tracy H. Reilly, MD

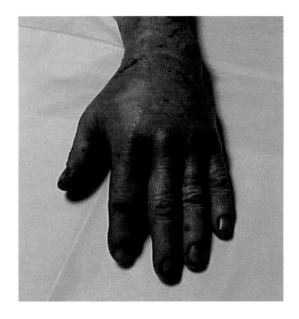

Case presentation: A 30-year-old automobile technician presents to the emergency department with a complaint of pain and swelling in the dorsum of his left hand near the metacarpal–phalangeal (MCP) joint of the index finger after injury with a grease injector. On exam there is slight swelling of the dorsum of the hand and a small pin-point puncture wound just proximal to the MCP joint of the index finger as noted in the picture. There is pain with passive movement, good capillary refill of the index finger and thumb, and no neurosensory deficits distal to the injury are appreciated.

Question: What is the most appropriate management?

A Check tetanus status, prescribe analgesics, and discharge home

B Prescribe antibiotics and analgesics, check tetanus status, and discharge home

C Obtain an X-ray, check tetanus status, immobilize with a splint, and discharge home with a prescription for antibiotics and analgesics and instructions to follow-up with an orthopedist in 3–5 days

D Obtain an X-ray, check tetanus status, and arrange an immediate surgical consultation for exploration and decompression debridement

E Insert a 14-gauge angiocatheter and aspirate the injected material

See page 117 for Answer, Diagnosis, and Discussion.

Case 62 | Chest pain in a middle-aged male patient with ST segment elevation

William J. Brady, MD

Case presentation: A 42-year-old male presented to the emergency department with chest pain. The examination revealed no distress with normal vital signs. A 12-lead electrocardiogram (ECG) is noted below. The patient received appropriate medications while laboratory studies and chest radiograph were performed; all such studies were within normal limits. Serial ECGs did not demonstrate a change in the ST segment elevation nor any further ST-segment or T-wave abnormality.

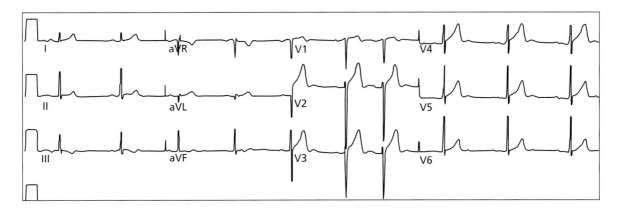

Question: The ECG pattern benign early repolarization is:
A Most often seen in elderly patients
B Indicative of underlying cardiac pathology
C A non-infarction cause of ST segment elevation
D Associated with an increased risk of sudden cardiac death
E Associated with valvular heart disease

See page 118 for Answer, Diagnosis, and Discussion.

Case 63 | Deformed globe following trauma

Joseph Robson, MD & Worth W. Everett, MD

Case presentation: A 79-year-old female was punched in the face during an assault and complains of pain and decreased vision in the left eye. On physical exam, there is minimal light perception on the left, and extraocular movement is decreased. Exam of the pupil is limited by blood in the anterior chamber. The deformity of her globe is shown right.

Question: Which of the following is the appropriate next step in the management of this patient?
A Access intraocular pressure
B Administer ocular steroids
C Discharge the patient with outpatient ophthalmology follow-up
D Administer anti-emetics, opioids, antibiotics, and call ophthalmologist for emergent consultation
E Perform emergent lateral canthotomy

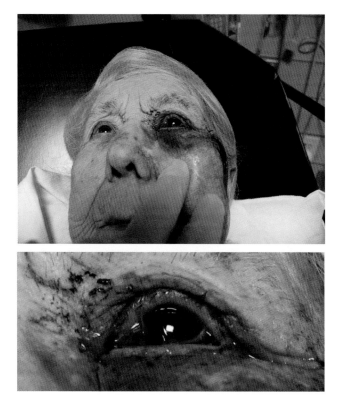

See page 119 for Answer, Diagnosis, and Discussion.

Case 64 | Adult male with atraumatic lower back pain and leg weakness

William J. Brady, MD

Case presentation: A 46-year-old male presented to the emergency department with lower back pain of 3 days duration. The patient denied trauma but noted previous back pain with a radicular distribution in the right lower extremity. The patient noted the recurrence of this pain with the onset of weakness in the legs. On examination, lower extremity weakness was noted in symmetric fashion, reduced sensation was found in the perineum, and the rectal examination demonstrated diminished tone. A post-void residual revealed 500 mL of urine remained in the bladder. Plain film radiographs were performed and demonstrated minimal degenerative change. Magnetic resonance imaging (MRI) of the lower spine was performed and is shown in the figure.

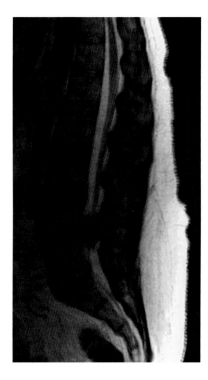

Question: What is the likely neurologic outcome of this clinical entity if appropriate medical care is offered immediately?

A Complete loss of motor and sensory function in the lower extremities

B Complete normalization of bowel and bladder function

C Normalization of motor function with progression of bladder dysfunction

D Stabilization of the current neurologic status without worsening

E Paraplegia

See page 120 for Answer, Diagnosis, and Discussion.

Case 65 | **Fever and rash in a child**

David L. Eldridge, MD

Case presentation: A 2-year-old male presents with a 6-day history of fever (temperatures up to 101°C and greater each day) and irritability. Accompanying this fever is the rash pictured. This rash is distributed along his face, trunk, and flexural surfaces of his extremities. He also has nonexudative conjunctivitis and dry, cracked, erythematous lips. With palpation of his neck, discover that he has a large (2.0 cm), firm, mobile, tender, left-sided anterior cervical lymph node. His hands and feet appear edematous.

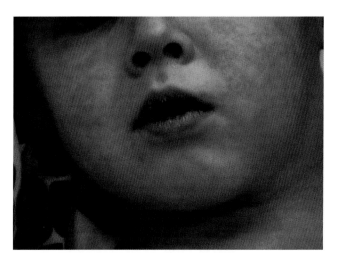

Question: Which of the following is associated with this clinical syndrome?

A Hemorrhagic gastritis

B Acute renal failure

C Intracranial abscess

D Coronary artery aneurysms

E Pancytopenia

See page 121 for Answer, Diagnosis, and Discussion.

Case 66 | **Yellow eyes and skin**

Jane M. Prosser, MD

Case presentation: A 48-year-old female presents to the emergency department with the chief complaint "My eyes are yellow." She denies having any other clinical complaints. Her physical exam is unremarkable except for what is pictured at right. No abdominal tenderness is elicited.

Question: Which of the following statements is true?
A Her scleral icterus effectively rules out hemolysis as a cause of her condition
B Scleral icterus is a more sensitive sign of hyperbilirubinemia than generalized jaundice
C The presence of Courvoisier's sign suggests an infectious etiology in this patient
D The lack of abdominal pain effectively rules out pancreatic cancer as a cause of her condition
E Vitamin A toxicity is a potential cause of this patient's condition

See page 122 for Answer, Diagnosis, and Discussion.

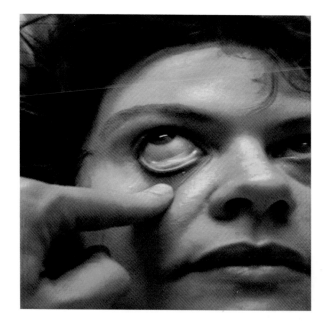

Case 67 | **Fishing in the stomach**

Christopher P. Holstege, MD

Case presentation: A 3-year-old male was playing with a lead fishing sinker. His mother was about to attempt to take it away from him when he suddenly began choking. By the time she reached her son, his choking had ceased and he was actively crying. He subsequently arrives at the emergency department asymptomatic. His physical exam is unremarkable, and an X-ray is obtained (see figure).

Question: Which of the following is the next most appropriate management step for this patient?
A Gastrointestinal lavage
B Endoscopic removal
C Whole bowel irrigation
D Activated charcoal administration
E. Syrup of ipecac administration

See page 122 for Answer, Diagnosis, and Discussion.

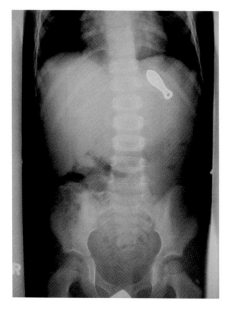

Case 68 | **Agitation in a botanist**

Alexander B. Baer, MD & Christopher P. Holstege, MD

Case presentation: A 32-year-old male botanist presents to the emergency department after paramedics received a call from his spouse that he was becoming markedly confused. According to his wife, this occurred after he drank a tea made from one of his plants, with the plant utilized noted below.

The patient is notably agitated, following no commands, constantly moving in the stretcher, picking relentlessly at the bed sheets, and talking with incomprehensible, mumbling

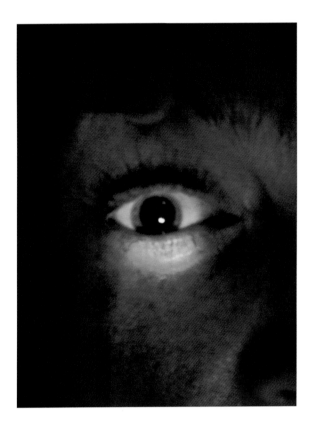

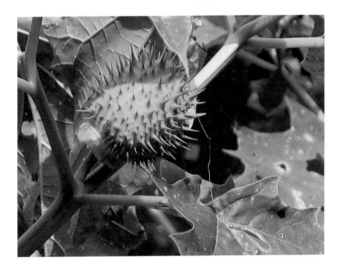

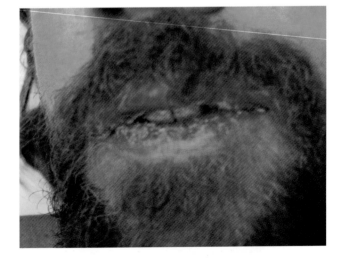

speech. The remainder of his examination is significant for the following: warm and dry to touch, no bowel sounds, pulse of 140 beats/minute, blood pressure of 160/90 mmHg, temperature of 38.4°C. An examination of his lips and pupils is noted (see figures above and left). A Foley is placed with return of 1.5 L of urine.

Question: Which of the following could produce this clinical syndrome?
A Jimson weed (*Datura stramonium*)
B Oleander (*Nerium oleander*)
C Lilly of the valley (*Convallaria majalis*)
D Monkshood (*Aconitum Napellus*)
E Death cap mushroom (*Amanita phalloides*)

See page 123 for Answer, Diagnosis, and Discussion.

Case 69 | **Skin target lesion**

Mara Becker, MD

Case presentation: A medical student rotating in emergency department comes for advice. She has developed a new rash on her calf over the past 24 hours. It is erythematous with central clearing and it has been expanding as the day progresses and is noted right. It is non-painful and non-pruritic. This is the only lesion she knows about thus far. She has had no fever and additionally only complains of some mild fatigue and muscle aches after hiking at Valley Forge in Pennsylvania on her last weekend off. She asks you if she should call out sick for her emergency department shift tonight.

Question: Which of the following is the next correct step in her management?

A Send her home with instructions to remain in isolation until the rash resolves
B Initiate therapy with doxycycline
C Perform incision and drainage at the center of the target lesion
D Administer brown recluse spider antivenom
E Infuse intravenous gammaglobulin

See page 124 for Answer, Diagnosis, and Discussion.

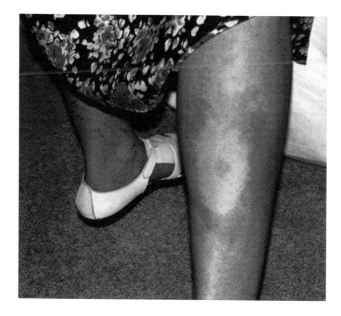

Case 70 | **Adult male with a sudden, severe headache**

Andrew L. Homer & William J. Brady, MD

Case presentation: A 55-year-old male presents to the emergency department complaining of the acute onset of a severe global headache while at rest 2 hours prior to presentation. The patient also complains of neck stiffness and nausea. Further history reveals the presence of milder headaches that have occurred intermittently over the past 2 weeks. His vitals are significant for a blood pressure of 165/95 mmHg and a pulse of 90 beats/minute; he is afebrile. The patient is in significant distress due to pain; the remainder of the examination is normal. While awaiting further evaluation, he suddenly becomes unresponsive. A head computerized tomography (CT) scan is performed emergently (see figure).

Question: Which of the following statements is true regarding this condition?

A Pressors should be administered to keep the mean systolic blood pressure above 160 mmHg

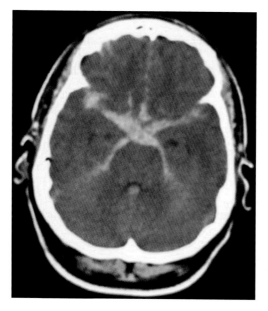

B Barbiturates are the antiseizure treatment of choice for this condition

C A classic "lucid interval" is present in one-third of patients who present early with this condition

D Lumbar puncture is the definitive treatment of choice for this patient

E A head CT may be falsely negative in as many as 10–15% of cases presenting early with headache

See page 125 for Answer, Diagnosis, and Discussion.

Case 71 | **Get them undressed!**

Munish Goyal, MD

Case presentation: A 19-year-old male is brought to the emergency department by his friends for fever and confusion. The patient is lethargic and warm to touch. His friends state he was complaining of a headache this morning and became increasingly confused today. He has no medical history and was asymptomatic yesterday. On exam, you note that he is hypotensive, tachycardic and has the following skin findings upon fully undressing him (see figure).

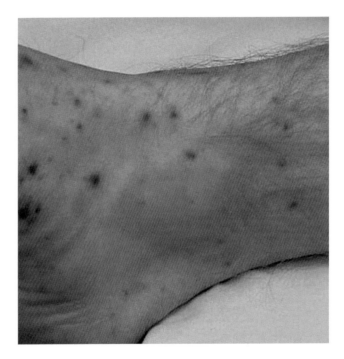

Question: What is the next most appropriate management strategy at this time?

A Administer acetaminophen and order a routine head computerized tomography scan to evaluate his headache

B Obtain a dermatology consultation

C Place the patient in isolation, administer immediate antibiotics, and draw appropriate cultures

D Order an electrocardiogram, alcohol level, electrolytes, and ammonia level to look for a source of his confusion

E Biopsy the skin lesion and send it to pathology

See page 125 for Answer, Diagnosis, and Discussion.

Case 72 | **Chest pain and subtle ST segment elevation**

William J. Brady, MD

Case presentation: A 46-year-old male presented to the emergency department with chest pain of 2 hours duration; the pain was accompanied by nausea and diaphoresis. The patient appeared pale and diaphoretic; otherwise, the examination was unremarkable. His electrocardiogram (ECG) was noted on the next page. The serum troponin was elevated, confirming the diagnosis of acute myocardial infarction (AMI). He was transferred to the catheterization laboratory for percutaneous coronary intervention. The patient had an uneventful hospital course.

Question: Choose the incorrect statement regarding reciprocal ST segment depression:

A Reciprocal ST segment depression is associated with an increased chance of poor outcome in ST-elevation myocardial infarction (STEMI)

B Reciprocal ST segment depression increases the probability that ST segment elevates results from AMI

C Reciprocal ST segment depression is defined as ST segment depression occurring in the STEMI patient

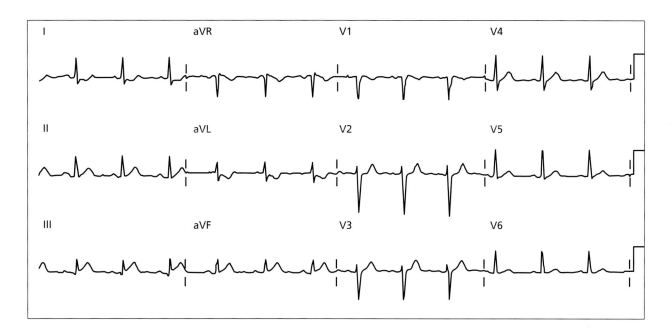

D Reciprocal ST segment depression includes the ST segment depression encountered in patients with confounding patterns such as left bundle branch block

E Reciprocal ST segment depression confers an improved prognosis

See page 126 for Answer, Diagnosis, and Discussion.

Case 73 | **Fluid in my eye**

Chris S. Bergstrom, MD & Alexander B. Baer, MD

Case presentation: A 22-year-old Caucasian male is evaluated in the emergency department with a complaint of marked left eye pain and blurred vision after being struck in the eye with a lead fishing weight. On physical exam, his visual acuity is 20/60 in the left eye. Pupillary examination is normal. Slit lamp exam shows a clear cornea. The anterior chamber is deep with suspended red blood cells in the aqueous humor (see figure). The iris detail is slightly obscured but otherwise normal with a central, round pupil.

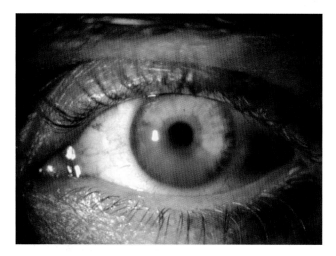

Question: What is the next best step in this patient's management?
A Administration of oral aspirin
B Infusion of intravenous heparin
C Emergent lateral canthotomy
D Administration of oral lisinopril
E Administration of atropine 1% ophthalmic drops

See page 126 for Answer, Diagnosis, and Discussion.

Case 74 | **Coma following head trauma**

Andrew L. Homer & William J. Brady, MD

Case presentation: A 19-year-male presents to the emergency department 30 minutes after a motor vehicle collision in which he sustained a head injury. Emergency medical services reports that he has no recollection of the accident and witnesses report that he was unconscious for approximately 1 minute. The patient is now alert and oriented to person, place, and time. He is complaining of only a headache at the site of impact. On exam, there is a 3 cm laceration on the left lateral forehead with an underlying bony step-off. The remainder of his physical exam is benign. Five minutes later, the patient becomes increasingly lethargic which progresses to a complete loss of consciousness. After stabilization, an emergent head computed tomography (CT) scan is ordered which is shown right.

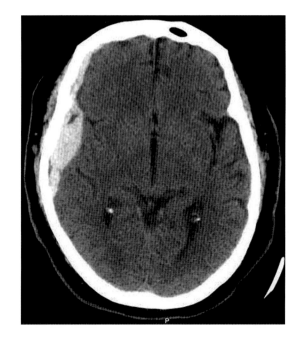

Question: Which of the following statements is true?
A A lucid interval is seen in over 90% of patients with this condition
B This condition is more common in the elderly
C Extravagated blood crosses suture lines in this condition
D Deaths are rare in patients with this condition if they are not in coma preoperatively
E Venous blood is most common source of the hematoma in this condition

See page 127 for Answer, Diagnosis, and Discussion.

Case 75 | **Blue hue following endoscopy**

Andrew L. Homer & Christopher P. Holstege, MD

Case presentation: A 39-year-old previously healthy female presents to the emergency department as a transfer from an outpatient endoscopy clinic. She had been in her usual state of health until 45 minutes into her esophagogastroduodenoscopy when she was noted to have a gradual decrease in her oxygen saturations and dyspnea. On arrival, her vital signs were as follows: pulse 125 beats/minute, blood pressure 96/43 mmHg, respiratory rate 36 breaths/minute, temperature 37.3°C. Her examination is unremarkable except for the skin findings shown in the figures (the patient's hand is on the right, the nurses hand is on the left). Her lungs are clear and her pulses are strong.

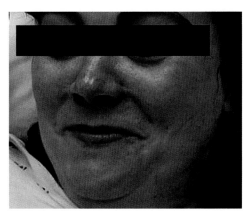

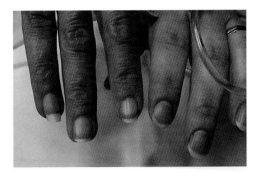

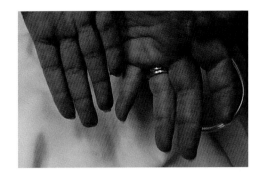

Question: Which of the following is the appropriate antidote for this toxicity?
A Prussian blue
B Physostigmine
C Deferoxamine
D Methylene blue
E Naloxone

See page 128 for Answer, Diagnosis, and Discussion.

Case 76 | Shoulder pain following direct blow

David F. Gaieski, MD

Case presentation: A 41-year-old male with no significant past medical history was playing touch football with friends at his college reunion. He was running with the ball, twisted sideways to try to avoid being tagged, and fell on the lateral aspect of his left shoulder with the right arm bent across the body. He experienced sudden onset of pain in his left shoulder and decreased range of motion. He denies numbness, tingling, or weakness in the arm. On examination, he is tender to palpation over his acromioclavicular joint, there are no breaks in his skin, and he has pain with forced adduction of the arm. He was given ibuprofen for pain control and an X-ray was obtained (see figure).

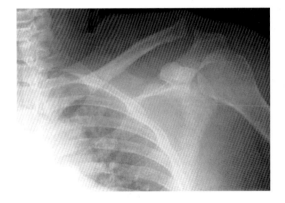

Question: The next most appropriate step in the management of this man's injury is:
A Orthopedic consultation for urgent surgical repair
B Figure eight wrap, pain control, and orthopedic follow-up
C Hematoma block and reduction
D Sling for immobilization and comfort, pain control, follow up with orthopedics
E Emergent computerized tomography (CT) scan of the shoulder

See page 129 for Answer, Diagnosis, and Discussion.

Case 77 | An overdose of prenatal vitamins

Christopher P. Holstege, MD & Adam K. Rowden, DO

Case presentation: A 16-year-old female intentionally overdosed on an unknown quantity of "vitamins." She arrives to the emergency department 4 hours after overdose complaining of nausea, vomiting, and epigastric abdominal pain.

Her initial vital signs reveal pulse 123 beats/minute, blood pressure 85/34 mmHg, respirations 24/minute, and temperature 37.2°C. Her examination is significant only for epigastric tenderness on palpation of her abdomen. Her laboratory studies are significant for the following: iron 567 mg/dL, serum bicarbonate 15 mEq/L, glucose 256 mg/dL, white blood count of 13.2×10^9/L. Her X-ray is pictured right.

Question: Which of the following is the next most appropriate management step for this patient?

A Begin an intravenous infusion of deferoxamine

B Administer dimercaprol (British Antilewisite, BAL) intramuscularly

C Infuse calcium disodium ethylenediaminetetraacetate (EDTA)

D Administer succimer (2,3-dimercaptosuccinic acid, DMSA) orally

E Administer D-penicillamine orally

See page 129 for Answer, Diagnosis, and Discussion.

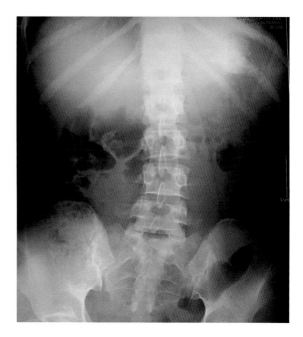

Case 78 | **Fever and rash in a child**

David L. Eldridge, MD

Case presentation: A 10-day-old male is brought to the emergency department by his mother. He has not eaten well for the past 24 hours and has reportedly been "very sleepy." Yesterday he began to develop a rash that now appears red at the base and is progressively "blistering" with clear fluid pictured below on his legs and face. He also has a swollen finger (right). Tonight he has had two episodes of uncontrollable shaking movements of his arms and legs – each lasting for a "few minutes." He was born 3 weeks premature and his mother claims no problems or issues with the pregnancy. He is afebrile but lethargic on exam currently.

Question: Which of the following tests would be *least helpful* in the clinical management of this patient given the likely diagnosis in this case?

A Computer tomography (CT) of the head

B Viral cultures of eyes, rectum, and skin lesions

C Polymerase chain reaction (PCR) testing of cerebrospinal fluid (CSF)

D Liver transaminase levels

E Chest radiograph

See page 131 for Answer, Diagnosis, and Discussion.

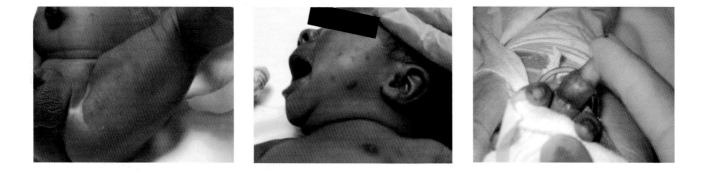

Case 79 | Lamp oil ingestion

David L. Eldridge, MD

Case presentation: A 2-year-old male was brought by ambulance to the emergency department. About 30 minutes before presentation, his mother had found him next to a soda bottle that contained lamp oil. The bottle was spilled all over the floor and she smelled lamp oil on his breath. The child was also coughing and choking. His mother called for an ambulance. Upon arrival, the emergency personnel found the child appearing sleepy, but with continued cough. On 2 L/minute of oxygen delivered by nasal cannula, his oxygen saturation was 89% with a respiratory rate of 55 breaths/minute. He had prominent subcostal retractions. Auscultation of his lungs revealed crackles bilaterally and decreased lung sounds at both bases.

The chest radiograph was taken one hour after the ingestion (see figure).

Question: Which of the following is most appropriate at this point in the management of this patient?
A Immediate gastric lavage as presentation is still within one hour of ingestion

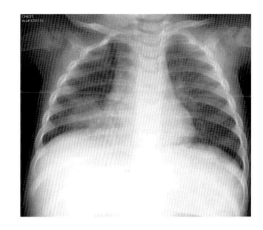

B Intravenous broad spectrum antibiotics given prophylactically
C Intravenous high-dose corticosteroids given prophylactically
D Continued close monitoring and supportive care
E Place nasogastric tube and give activated charcoal

See page 131 for Answer, Diagnosis, and Discussion.

Case 80 | Diffuse ankle pain following a fall

Andrew D. Perron, MD & Christopher T. Bowe, MD

Case presentation: A 21-year-old male patient presents to the emergency department with ankle and foot pain after jumping to the ground from a height of approximately 10 feet. He is unable to ambulate due to pain. Examination revealed medial ankle pain over the deltoid ligament on the medial ankle. Neurovascular examination was normal. A radiograph was performed (see figure).

Question: In this patient with an axial load mechanism, palpable medial ankle tenderness, and the radiograph that is shown, what emergency department management course should be pursued?
A Ace wrap, ice, elevation, and discharge home
B Aircast, weight bearing as tolerated, and discharge home
C Splint, crutches, and primary care outpatient follow-up
D Potential further imaging (i.e. computerized axial tomography scan) and orthopedic consultation
E Hematoma block and fracture reduction

See page 132 for Answer, Diagnosis, and Discussion.

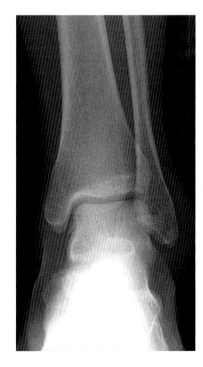

Case 81 | **Emergency department drop-off**

Tracy H. Reilly, MD

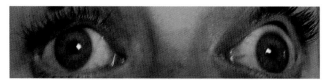

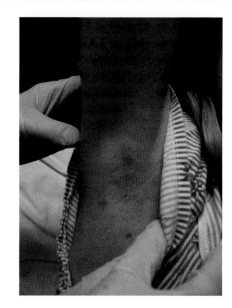

Case presentation: A 22-year-old college student is dropped off by her friends in the triage area of the emergency department after the friends told the triage nurse that the patient would not wake up. The patient is lethargic, is arousable only to painful stimuli and is without obvious signs of trauma. The presenting vital signs are: pulse 52 beats/minute, blood pressure of 85/70 mmHg, respirations 8/minute and shallow, oxygen saturation 90% on room air, and temperature 36°C. The remainder of the patient's examination is unremarkable except for the eye exam and the skin exam noted under the axilla (see figures).

Question: Which of the following signs or symptoms would least likely be observed in a patient suspected of an acute opioid overdose?
A Respiratory depression
B Miosis
C Somnolence
D Bradycardia
E Hyperthermia

See page 133 for Answer, Diagnosis, and Discussion.

Case 82 | **Weakness and bradycardia in an elderly female patient**

William J. Brady, MD

Case presentation: A 78-year-old woman with a history of coronary artery disease experienced progressive weakness associated with chest pain. On arrival in the emergency department, the patient was without distress. The vital signs were significant only for bradycardia with a rate of 55 beats/minute (bpm). The 12-lead electrocardiogram (ECG) demonstrated sinus bradycardia at a rate of 62 bpm with inferior ST segment depression; a bedside qualitative test was positive for troponin. The patient was diagnosed with a non-ST elevation myocardial infarction (STEMI) while appropriate therapy was initiated. Approximately 45 minutes after arrival, the patient developed hypotension with profound weakness and recurrent chest

pain. The blood pressure was 85 mmHg by palpation and the pulse was approximately 25 bpm. The ECG monitor demonstrated the rhythm below.

Question: The most frequent etiology of this type of rhythm is:
A Acute myocardial infarction
B Cardiotoxic medication ingestion
C Acute myocarditis
D Primary conduction system disease
E Pericarditis

See page 133 for Answer, Diagnosis, and Discussion.

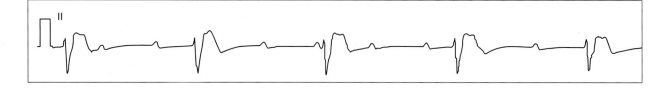

Case 83 | **Blurred vision following yard work**

Allyson Kreshak, MD

Case presentation: A 46-year-old male presented with a chief complaint of blurry vision. The patient had been outside cleaning up his yard in Central Virginia prior to developing the symptoms. He denied headache, nausea, or vomiting and had no other neurologic complaints. He denied a history of trauma. He was otherwise healthy. His vital signs were as follows: heart rate 88 beats/minute, blood pressure 142/76 mmHg, oral temperature 37.1°C, respirations 16/minute, pulse oximetry 99% on room air. His exam was remarkable for only the finding noted in the figure.

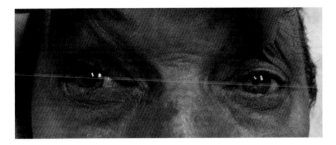

Question: Which of the following is a likely cause of this patient's condition?

A Stroke

B Tentorial herniation

C Cataracts

D Tonic pupil

E Jimson weed exposure (*Datura stramonium*)

See page 134 for Answer, Diagnosis, and Discussion.

Case 84 | **A gagging child**

Maureen Chase, MD & Worth W. Everett, MD

Case presentation: The mother of a 3-year-old boy presents to the emergency department with her son who refuses to eat today and gagged on the few bites of dinner he tried last night. She noted some mild drooling today but reports that he has otherwise been active and playful. She expresses concern that he may have swallowed something while playing unsupervised for a brief period yesterday afternoon. The child is well-appearing with normal phonation and no

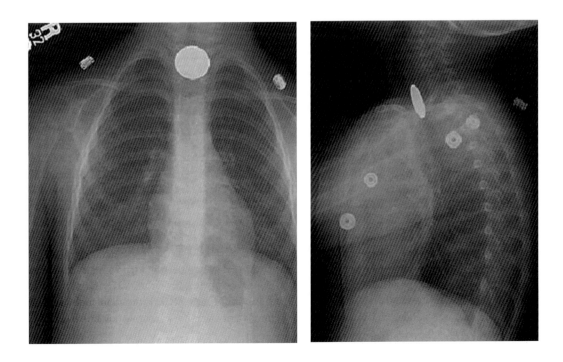

stridor. The remainder of his physical exam is unremarkable. Obtain the radiographs pictured on page 53.

Question: What is the next most appropriate management strategy?
A Order a computerized tomography (CT) scan of the neck
B Consult an ear-nose-throat (ENT) specialist for an emergent nasopharyngeal laryngoscopy
C Attempt to see if the child can drink and, if so, discharge home with repeat X-ray in 24 hours to determine if the object has passed
D Consult gastroenterology for emergent esophagoscopy
E Emergently intubate the child for airway protection

See page 135 for Answer, Diagnosis, and Discussion.

Case 85 | **A child with bruises of different ages**

David L. Eldridge, MD

Case presentation: The 3-year-old male pictured right is brought in by his parents because of altered mental status following a fall. His parents report that about an hour ago, he tripped on some of his own toys and fell down the stairs at home. He did not lose consciousness but he has been "very sleepy" since. On exam he is lethargic but arousable and obeys commands. He also has gross deformity, point tenderness, and erthyema at the middle anterior aspect of his right humerus. He also has facial contusions and back contusions as pictured that appear to be of varying ages.

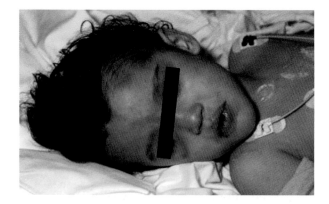

Question: Which of the following bruising patterns is least concerning for child abuse?
A Bruising on the right knee of a 2-month-old infant
B Multiple bruising on the knees and shins of a developmentally appropriate 3 year old
C A developmentally normal 5-year-old child with multiple bruising along his cheeks and forehead
D A developmentally normal 2 year old with bruising along the arms that appears to have a consistent loop pattern
E Multiple bruises along the buttocks of a developmentally normal 2-year-old child

See page 136 for Answer, Diagnosis, and Discussion.

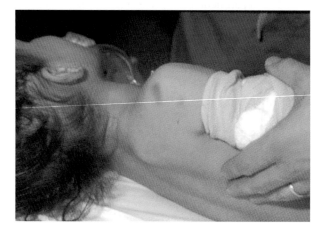

Case 86 | **Traumatic eye pain and proptosis**

Chris S. Bergstrom, MD & Alexander B. Baer, MD

Case presentation: A 32-year-old female is seen in the emergency department after a domestic altercation. She is complaining of left eye pain, swelling, and decreased vision. Ocular examination reveals visual acuity of 20/400 in the left eye with limited extraocular motility. An afferent pupillary defect is present in the left eye. There is marked proptosis of the left eye with periorbital edema and bullous subconjunctival hemorrhage as noted in the picture. The globe is hard and there is resistance to retropulsion. The intraocular pressure is 65 mmHg in the left eye.

Question: Which of the following is not indicated in the treatment of this condition?

A Timolol
B Brimonidine
C Acetazolamide
D Lateral canthotomy
E Lisinopril

See page 136 for Answer, Diagnosis, and Discussion.

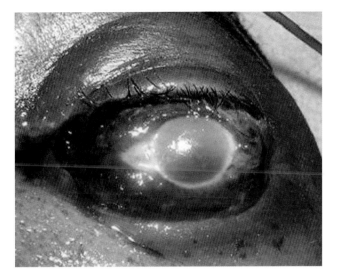

Case 87 | **Post-prandial abdominal pain in an elderly woman**

Hoi Lee, MD

Case presentation: A 70-year-old woman presents to the emergency department with a one-week history of progressive abdominal pain and intermittent vomiting. She had a previous history of bloating and intermittent post-prandial abdominal pain. She has never had surgery. On examination, the abdomen is mildly distended and tympanitic, has normal bowel sounds, and is moderately tender to palpation in right upper quadrant. Abdominal X-rays show distended loops of small bowel and gas within the liver in a branching pattern. Abdominal computed tomography (CT) scan with intravenous and oral contrast reveals the image shown right.

Question: Which of the following is true regarding this condition?

A Less than one-third of patients with this condition have a previous history of biliary symptoms, and overall mortality is less than 1%
B This condition accounts for less than 5% of all non-strangulated small bowel obstructions seen in the general population
C Its diagnosis prompts outpatient follow-up with a surgical consultation
D Plain abdominal X-ray is usually sufficient to make the diagnosis

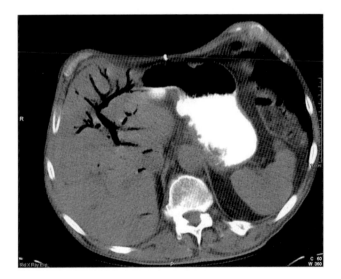

E *Rigler's Triad* consists of large bowel obstruction, pneumobilia, and adhesions of the large bowel

See page 137 for Answer, Diagnosis, and Discussion.

Case 88 | **Hyperthermia, tachycardia, and confusion in a teenager**

Alexander B. Baer, MD

Case presentation: An 18-year-old South American male was traveling from Miami to New York City by Amtrak train. While at a train station along the way, he was noted by the conductor to be acting oddly and the police were called. On search of his possessions, the packets pictured below were discovered.

He was subsequently transported by paramedics with police escort to the emergency department. His initial vital signs on presentation are as follows: blood pressure 195/113 mmHg, pulse 143 beats/minute, respirations 36/minute, temperature 38.7°C. His examination is significant for confusion, agitation, mydriasis, diaphoresis, and tremor. A radiograph of his abdomen is noted below.

Question: Which of the following would be indicated in his management?
A Propranolol
B Lorazepam
C Sotalol
D Procainamide
E Gastric lavage

See page 137 for Answer, Diagnosis, and Discussion.

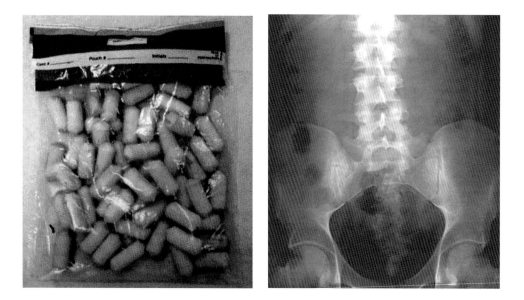

Case 89 | **Acute onset double vision**

Chris S. Bergstrom, MD & Alexander B. Baer, MD

Case presentation: A 47-year-old female presents to the emergency department with a complaint of acute retro-bulbar pain and left lid droop. She also states that when she holds her eyelid open she has double vision. Her past medical and ocular history is negative for hypertension and diabetes. She takes no medications. Physical examination reveals a complete ptosis of the left upper lid as noted in the figure.

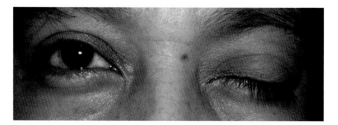

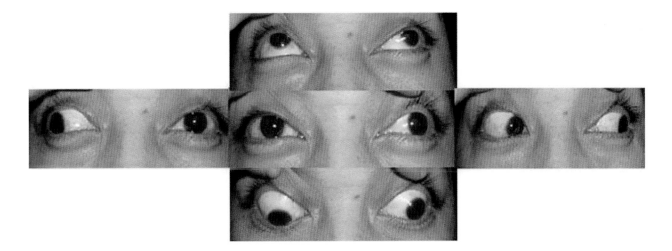

Manually lifting the eyelid reveals the left eye with an outward deviation. Evaluation pictured of the extraocular muscles shows marked reduction in adduction, elevation, and depression of the left globe.

Visual acuity is 20/20 in each eye. Pupillary testing shows marked anisocoria with the right pupil 3 mm and the left pupil 8 mm. The left pupil does not constrict to light stimulation. The remaining ocular and neurological examination is normal.

Question: What is the most likely cause of this patient's physical exam?
A Bell's palsy
B Forth cranial nerve palsy
C Third cranial nerve palsy
D Benign strabismus of childhood
E Fifth cranial nerve palsy

See page 138 for Answer, Diagnosis, and Discussion.

Case 90 | **Ankle pain and inability to walk**

Christopher T. Bowe, MD

Case presentation: A 32-year-old male patient presents to the emergency department after sustaining a fall while walking down an incline. He reported a twisting motion of his left ankle and an inability to stand on his left leg since the fall. He denies other injury. Radiographs were preformed and are noted below.

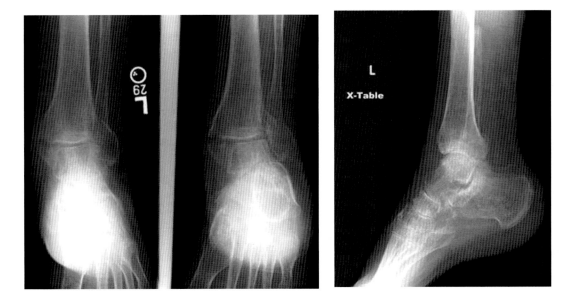

Question: In the patient with the injury noted on the radiographs, how can the injury be best described and initially managed?

A Nondisplaced fracture – splint with outpatient orthopedic follow-up

B Fracture/dislocation – reduction and splint with outpatient orthopedic follow-up

C Unstable bimalleolar fracture – urgent orthopedic consultation

D Unstable trimalleolar fracture – urgent orthopedic consultation

E Stable bimalleolar fracture – splint with outpatient orthopedic follow-up

See page 139 for Answer, Diagnosis, and Discussion.

Case 91 | Tongue swelling in a hypertensive female

Kevin S. Barlotta, MD & Alexander B. Baer, MD

Case presentation: A 60-year-old female with a history of hypertension presents to the emergency department with a complaint of progressive tongue swelling over the past 8 hours. She denies having eaten anything new or atypical, there is no history of an insect envenomation, and she has had no new medication changes. She denies having difficulty breathing and is able to swallow her secretions. She is only taking 1 prescription medication for her hypertension: lisinopril. She reports one previous episode one week ago of less severity that spontaneously resolved. Her examination is significant for marked tongue edema noted in the picture with the inability to fully retract the tongue back into the mouth. The rest of her examination is unremarkable.

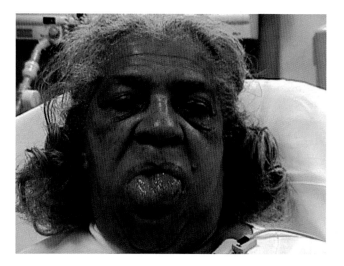

Question: What is the next most appropriate management strategy at this time?

A Reassurance and discharge to home with a prescription for a first generation cephalosporin

B Emergent dentistry consultation, obtain blood cultures, and administer a third generation cephalosporin

C Admission to a monitored unit for observation, cessation of her lisinopril, antihistamines, and corticosteroids.

D Computerized tomography (CT) scan of the neck with intravenous contrast to evaluate for abscess and consultation with ear-nose-throat service for emergent incision and drainage

E Chest CT to evaluate for a potential lesion obstructing venous drainage from the head through the superior vena cava

See page 140 for Answer, Diagnosis, and Discussion.

Case 92 | Wide complex tachycardia in an older male patient

William J. Brady, MD

Case presentation: A 57-year-old male with a history of angina and coronary artery disease experienced a sudden syncopal event. The patient regained consciousness minutes later and noted only palpitations and weakness. He was transported to the emergency department via private vehicle. On arrival, he was pale and diaphoretic with a blood pressure of 80 mmHg by palpation and a pulse of 190 beats/minute. The cardiac monitor below demonstrated a wide complex tachycardia as showed in leads II and V. The patient was sedated and cardioverted with the return of sinus rhythm and an adequate blood pressure.

Question: In the setting of a wide complex tachycardia, select the correct statement:

A Urgent therapy is dependent upon a precise rhythm diagnosis

B Ventricular tachycardia and supraventricular tachycardia with aberrant conduction are easily distinguished

C Certain electrocardiographic features suggest the diagnosis of ventricular tachycardia

D Patient age is an absolute indicator of rhythm diagnosis in a wide complex tachycardia

E Wide complex tachycardia due to drugs is easily distinguished from other causes

See page 141 for Answer, Diagnosis, and Discussion.

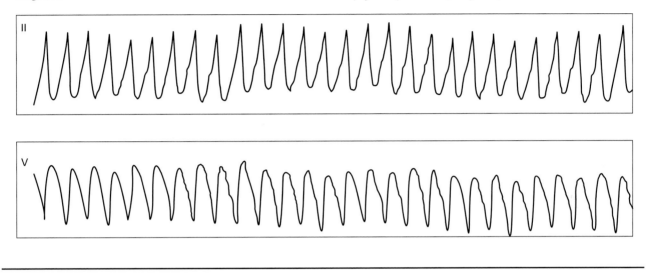

Case 93 | **Acute onset double vision**

Chris S. Bergstrom, MD & Alexander B. Baer, MD

Case presentation: A 37-year-old male is seen in the emergency department with a complaint of blurred vision, redness, and foreign body sensation in the right eye. His symptoms started 3 days prior to presentation when he felt something hit his eye while working under his car. His visual acuity is 20/60 in the right eye and the pupillary examination is normal. The conjunctiva is injected and there is a central, metallic corneal foreign body embedded 30% into the corneal stroma with an associated rust ring and infiltrate (as pictured). There is 1+ cellular reaction in the anterior chamber. The iris and lens are normal.

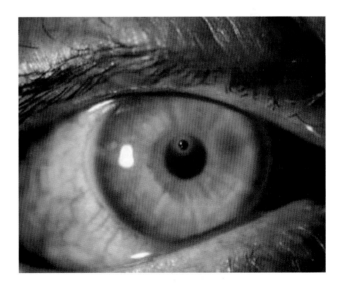

Question: What is the next most appropriate step in the management of this patient?

A Magnetic resonance imaging of the eye to rule out intraorbital foreign body

B Intraorbital injection of lidocaine prior to manipulation of the foreign body

C Eye irrigation and then discharge to home with outpatient ophthalmology reevaluation in 1 week

D Eye patch, antibiotics, and follow-up with the patient's primary physician in 3–5 days

E Removal of the ocular foreign body under topical anesthesia using a 25 g needle

See page 142 for Answer, Diagnosis, and Discussion.

Case 94 | **Foot pain in a gymnast**

Hoi Lee, MD

Case presentation: A 19-year-old female gymnast presents with worsening pain in her right foot that developed over the previous 3 days. The pain is located over the lateral aspect of her foot. Physical examination reveals mild tenderness with palpation over the fifth metatarsal with associated swelling in the area. Patient is able to ambulate with a slight limp. Her foot radiographs are shown.

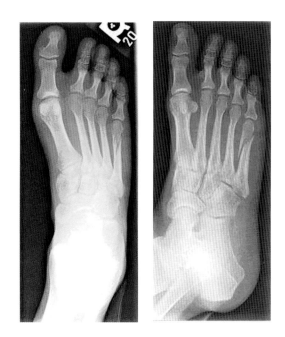

Question: Which of the following is true regarding this injury?

A A computed axial tomography (CT) scan should be obtained to rule out possible metatarsophalangeal joint involvement

B Nonunion due to lack of vascular supply is a common complication for this fracture

C Treatment includes application of a short-leg walking cast for up to 4–6 weeks, and outpatient follow-up with an orthopedist

D Emergent orthopedic consultation is required for this type of injury

E Hematoma block with fracture reduction should be performed

See page 144 for Answer, Diagnosis, and Discussion.

Case 95 | **New facial droop**

Andrew D. Perron, MD & Christopher T. Bowe, MD

Case presentation: A 43-year-old female presents to the emergency department with a concern that she is having a stroke. She notes left facial weakness, pain in her left ear, and that whenever she drinks water it spills out the left side of her mouth. The symptoms have progressed over the past 24 hours. The photograph demonstrates the patient when she is asked to "smile and look up".

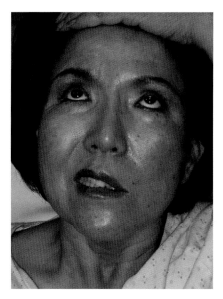

Question: In a patient with this condition, which of the following medical treatments should be considered?

A Prednisone

B Gamma globulin

C Thrombolytics

D Heparin

E Edrophonium

See page 145 for Answer, Diagnosis, and Discussion.

Case 96 | **Eye pain and swelling**

Adam K. Rowden, DO & Chris S. Bergstrom, MD

Case presentation: A 25-year-old, previously healthy female presents with a complaint of eye pain for 3 days. She denies associated fever or chills. She has no change in her vision. She denies nasal discharge or sinus pressure. She initially noted redness of her eyelid which then progressively swelled and became more painful. Her physical exam (noted in the picture) reveals her eyelid and surrounding soft tissue to be warm and swollen. Her extra-ocular movements are intact; her visual acuity is normal; her pupillary reflex is intact; the conjunctiva is non-inflamed. Her vitals are normal and she is afebrile.

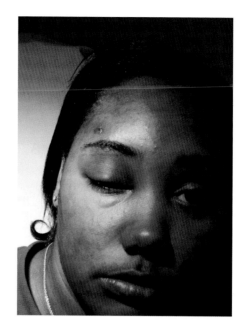

Question: Which of the following is the next correct step in her management?

A Administer oral antibiotics to cover *S. aureus* and discharge her home with close outpatient follow-up with her primary care physician

B Administer intravenous antibiotics to cover *H. influenzae* and admit to the hospital

C Administer intravenous antibiotics to cover *H. influenzae* and *S. aureus*, and obtain an enhanced orbital CT

D Obtain an urgent ear-nose-throat (ENT) consultation for debridement and start intravenous antibiotics

E Initiate high-dose prednisone and send an erythrocyte sedimentation rate (ESR) while arranging rheumatology follow-up

See page 146 for Answer, Diagnosis, and Discussion.

Case 97 | **Shortening and rotation of the leg following trauma**

Jane M. Prosser, MD

Case presentation: A 34-year-old male is brought by helicopter to the emergency department after involvement in a motor vehicle crash. The medics report significant damage to the car requiring extrication of the patient. The patient is awake and alert. He complains of severe pain in his left lower extremity but denies other complaints. His external examination is noted in the figure and his pulses and sensation are intact in both lower extremities.

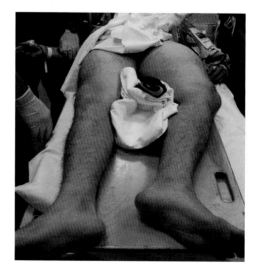

Question: Which of the following statements is true?

A This patient likely has an isolated lower extremity injury

B An emergent orthopedics consult should be obtained prior to completion of a trauma evaluation

C Lower extremity angiography should be performed immediately

D This patient could have a femoral shaft fracture in addition to a hip fracture

E Immediate hematoma block and fracture reduction should be performed

See page 147 for Answer, Diagnosis, and Discussion.

Case 98 | **Spider bite in the night**

Adam K. Rowden, DO & Christopher P. Holstege, MD

Case presentation: A 25-year-old female presents to the emergency department with severe back pain and spasm. She also complains of nausea and chest tightness. She was awoken from sleep by a "pin-prick" sensation to her right thigh. A search of her bed sheets revealed the creature pictured. Over the next 60 minutes, her pain intensified first in her right leg, and then into her groin and into her back. She took ibuprofen without relief. Her physical exam is significant for a red target lesion approximately 1 cm in circumference on her right thigh, hypertension (180/100 mmHg), tachycardia (145 beats/minute), and marked spasm of her lumbar and thoracic paraspinal muscles.

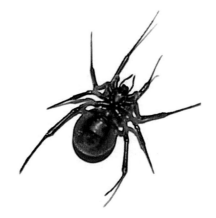

Question: Which of the following is most appropriate initial therapy?

A Start an infusion of intravenous calcium chloride through her hand line

B Immediately push antivenin intravenously

C Administer intravenous nitrates and beta blockers for her marked tachycardia and hypertension

D Administer intravenous opioids for pain control and benzodiazepines for muscle relaxation

E Apply a lymphatic tourniquet to prevent further systemic absorption of the venom

See page 148 for Answer, Diagnosis, and Discussion.

Case 99 | **Wide complex tachycardia in a young adult**

William J. Brady, MD

Case presentation: A 24-year-old female patient with no medical history of significance was transported to the emergency department via paramedics complained of sudden weakness and palpitations; all symptoms had resolved prior to the paramedic's arrival at the scene. In the emergency department, the patient noted recurrence of the symptoms; examination at that time demonstrated an alert patient with minimal distress. The vital signs were blood pressure

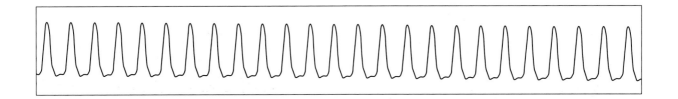

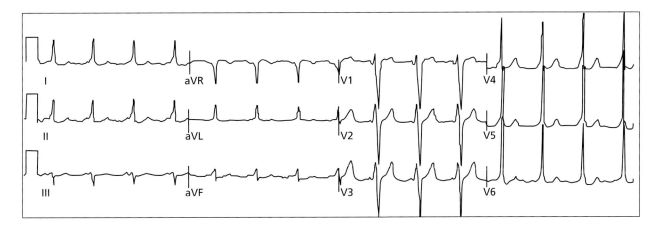

100/70 mmHg, pulse 240 beats/minute, and respiration 38/minute. The monitor revealed a rapid, wide complex rhythm noted in the figure on page 62.

The patient received amiodarone intravenously; during the infusion, she became lethargic with a sudden reduction in blood pressure. Immediate electrical cardioversion was undertaken with return of a normal mental status and the electrocardiogram noted above; the remainder of the examination normalized as well.

Question: Of the listed interventions, the most appropriate initial intervention is:

A Intravenous diltiazem

B Oral metoprolol

C Intravenous procainamide

D Oral amiodarone

E Intravenous potassium

See page 149 for Answer, Diagnosis, and Discussion.

Case 100 | **Abdominal pain in a trauma victim**

Esther H. Chen, MD

Case presentation: A 25-year-old male unrestrained driver involved in a head-on collision with another vehicle presents with a complaint of chest pain and abdominal pain.

There was no airbag deployment and the car was moderately damaged. Vital signs are blood pressure 95/60 mmHg, pulse 120 beats/minute, respiratory rate 20/minute, oxygen

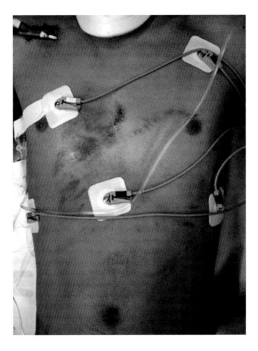

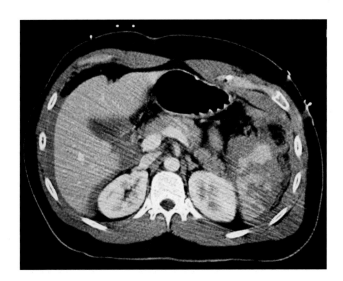

saturation 100% on room air. The exam is significant for the skin finding noted in the figure, crepitus over the left lateral chest wall, and left upper quadrant abdominal tenderness.

Question: Which statement is true regarding this injury?
A These injuries always require operative repair
B The liver, not the spleen, is more commonly injured after blunt abdominal trauma
C Patients with an initial negative computerized axial tomography (CT) scan can still develop delayed splenic rupture 1 week after the initial injury

D A focused assessment by sonography in trauma (FAST) ultrasound exam is the most accurate for identifying abdominal solid organ injury
E Greater than 90% of splenic injuries are associated with rib fractures

See page 150 for Answer, Diagnosis, and Discussion.

Part 2 | **Answers, Diagnoses, and Discussion**

Case 1 | **Rash following brush fire**

Answer: B

Diagnosis: Poison ivy dermatitis

Discussion: Poison ivy is a plant contained within the species *Toxicodendron* (Figure 1.1). This species includes poison ivy, poison oak, and poison sumac. The *Toxicodendron* species contains a substance called urushiol. In susceptible individuals, urushiol triggers a type IV delayed hypersensitivity reaction. The most common reaction seen involves the skin following direct contact with the plant (Figure 1.2). However, if a susceptible person is exposed to smoke from burning plants, not only is a skin reaction seen, but also the eyes, airway, and lungs may be involved. Lesions generally appear within 12–48 hours, although they may appear earlier. New lesions may continue to appear for up to a month. Initially, these lesions tend to occur from the slow reaction to adsorbed urushiol; however, lesions that appear later are often secondary to contact with contaminated surfaces (i.e. contaminated clothing and pet hair). The fluid from the vesicles of a rash does not contain urushiol and is not an irritant source for new lesions.

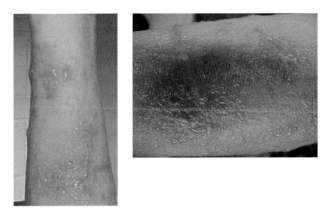

Figure 1.2 Classic *Toxicodendron* dermatitis of the arm following direct skin contact with the plant.

Urushiol penetrates the skin and binds within 15 minutes of contact. If the toxin can be removed before this occurs, the reaction can be avoided. Copious water irrigation should be performed if contact has occurred. Contaminated clothes should be washed. Topical preparations for symptomatic relief include Domeboro™, calamine, and oatmeal baths. Oral antihistamines (i.e. hydroxyzine) are of benefit for the relief of pruritus. Oral systemic steroids are the standard for severe toxicodendron associated dermatitis. Prednisone or methylprednisolone can be administered and should be tapered over no less than 10–14 days. Early withdrawal of steroid therapy can lead to a return of the rash. Oral analgesics occasionally are required in the worst cases.

Further reading

1 Guin JD. Treatment of toxicodendron dermatitis (poison ivy and poison oak). *Skin Therapy Lett* 2001;**6**(7):3–5.
2 Lee NP, Arriola ER. Poison ivy, oak, and sumac dermatitis. *West J Med* 1999;**171**(5–6):354–5.

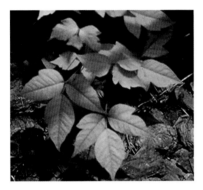

Figure 1.1 Poison ivy.

Case 2 | **Herbalist with bradycardia and vision changes**

Answer: A

Diagnosis: Cardiac glycoside toxicity due to foxglove ingestion

Discussion: The cardiac glycosides are potent cardiovascular agents that include digoxin and digitoxin. Several plants, including oleander (*Nerium oleander*), foxglove (*Digitalis purpurea*), and lily of the valley (*Convallaria majalis*), contain the cardiac glycosides. In this case, the patient was chronically ingesting foxglove as an herbal remedy and subsequently developed cardiac glycoside toxicity with hyperkalemia and a junctional bradycardia. The glycosides slow conduction through the atrioventricular (AV) node. When present at toxic levels, these agents impair conduction while increasing automaticity – most often producing ectopic rhythms at rapid rates. The signs and symptoms of cardiac glycoside intoxication depend on whether the poisoning is acute or chronic. In an acute ingestion, nausea and vomiting are prominent along with hyperkalemia and cardiotoxicity manifested by dysrhythmias. In chronic intoxication, nonspecific symptoms such as malaise, weakness, and visual disturbances may be encountered, as well as cardiac dysrhythmias.

A broad range of cardiac dysrhythmias is seen in the patient with cardiac glycoside toxicity, including bradycardia, AV block, and tachycardia. The three classically described dysrhythmias which suggest the diagnosis include paroxysmal atrial tachycardia with block, junctional tachycardia, and ventricular tachycardia. Paroxysmal atrial tachycardia with block occurs progressively rather than suddenly; in fact, the term "paroxysmal" is a misnomer. The atrial rate is usually between 150 and 250 beats per minute; the degree of AV block varies, with second degree and Wenckebach being the most common forms.

Junctional rhythms, including junctional tachycardia, result from suppression of impulse formation at the sinoatrial node to the degree that the inherent AV pacemaker cells outpace the sinoatrial nodal cells. The escape rhythms result in a regular ventricular rate of 40–60 beats per minute, but accelerated junctional rhythms and junctional bradycardias are common. Ventricular tachycardia is a common manifestation of severe cardiac glycoside poisoning. As a result of increased automaticity, premature ventricular beats are often the earliest dysrhythmia associated with cardiac glycoside intoxication and account for half of the dysrhythmias associated with digitalis. Bidirectional ventricular tachycardia is a rare dysrhythmia which is most commonly caused by cardiac glycoside toxicity.

Potential treatment for symptomatic patients with cardiac glycoside toxicity includes the administration of digoxin-specific Fab fragments. For coexisting hyperkalemia, the early administration of intravenous crystalloids, albuterol, sodium bicarbonate, and insulin with glucose should be performed to help decrease the hyperkalemia.

Further reading

1 Ma G, Brady WJ, Pollack M, Chan TC. Electrocardiographic manifestations: digitalis toxicity. *J Emerg Med* 2001;**20**: 145–52.

2 Rich SA, Libera JM, Locke RJ. Treatment of foxglove extract poisoning with digoxin-specific Fab fragments. *Ann Emerg Med* 1993;**22**(12):1904–7.

3 Holstege CP, Eldridge DL, Rowden A. Electrocardiographic changes associated with poisoning. *Emerg Med Clin North Am* 2006;**24**(1): 159–77.

Case 3 | **Acute eye pain and blurred vision in an elderly female**

Answer: C

Diagnosis: Acute angle closure glaucoma

Discussion: Acute angle closure glaucoma is much rarer than open angle glaucoma. It generally affects patients in their sixth to seventh decade of life and is slightly more common in females. Acute angle closure glaucoma is characterized by a rapid rise in intraocular pressure. The rapid increase in pressure causes conjunctival injection and corneal edema as shown in the photo on page 4. The major factor responsible for precipitating an angle closure attack is prolonged periods of mid-pupillary dilation. Acute angle closure attacks tend to occur after prolonged periods in dim illumination. Attacks also occur after periods of severe stress due to adrenergic stimulation and dilation of the pupil. Both adrenergic agonists and anticholinergic agents, either topical or systemic, are also capable of precipitating an acute attack. The intraocular pressure rises when the iris occludes the trabecular meshwork preventing aqueous outflow. Severe pressure elevations can occur within 1 hour resulting in permanent damage.

Initial management of acute angle closure glaucoma involves pharmacologic lowering of the intraocular pressure by inhibiting aqueous production. A careful medical history should be taken, specifically for asthma, chronic obstructive pulmonary disease, congestive heart failure, renal failure, and drug allergies. If not contraindicated, a topical beta blocker such as timolol or levobunolol, 0.5%, should be instilled along with topical brimonidine 0.15%. A carbonic anhydrase inhibitor such as acetazolamide, two 250 mg tablets, should be given orally or 500 mg given intravenously. Severe cases may require intravenous mannitol, in doses of 1–2 g/kg infused over 45 minutes. Vital signs should be monitored closely when giving mannitol. The intraocular pressure should be rechecked within 1 hour. Ophthalmologic consultation is necessary for patients with acute angle closure glaucoma since the definitive treatment is a peripheral laser iridectomy.

Further reading

1 Saw SM, Gazzard G, Friedman DS. Interventions for angle-closure glaucoma: an evidence-based update. *Ophthalmology* 2003;**110**(10):1869–78.

2 Tripathi RC, Tripathi BJ, Haggerty C. Drug-induced glaucomas: mechanism and management. *Drug Saf* 2003;**26**(11):749–67.

Case 4 | **Suspicious hand pain**

Answer: C

Diagnosis: Boxer's fracture

Discussion: Fractures of the 5th metacarpal neck are among the most common fractures in the hand, accounting for 10% of all hand fractures. These fractures are often caused by striking a solid object with a closed fist and are known as a "boxer's fracture." However, this is a misnomer since these fractures rarely occur during boxing. Rather, a skilled fighter may fracture the index metacarpal because the blow comes straight from the body along the line of greatest force transmission, while an inexperienced fighter may use a "roundhouse" type motion to cause this injury.

Typically, metacarpal neck fractures will have an apex dorsal angulation (palmar angulation of the distal fragment). Maintaining the fracture in reduction can be difficult due to deforming forces of the surrounding muscles. Metacarpal neck fractures rarely require surgery. Minimally angulated or displaced fractures can be managed with simple immobilization for 3–4 weeks. The degree of acceptable angulation is controversial. Most surgeons agree that no more than 45° of angulation is allowed in the 5th metacarpal. Some authors argue that 5th metacarpal neck fractures with any degree of angulation do not need reduction and may simply be immobilized for 4 weeks. The reasoning behind this is that simple immobilization will not maintain satisfactory reduction. However, rotational injury does need to be addressed as this can impair function and result in a deformity with an overlap of the affected and adjacent fingers. If the decision is to reduce, the most common method of reduction is the *90–90 method*. After anesthesia (a hematoma block), traction is applied to the metacarpal distal to the injury. The metacarpal-phalangeal and interphalangeal joints are then flexed at 90° and pressure is applied volarly over the metacarpal shaft and dorsally over the flexed proximal interphalangeal (PIP) joint.

The decision to reduce or simply immobilize should be made by an experienced emergency physician or in conjunction

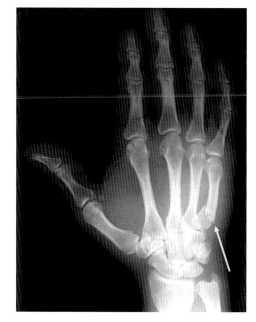

Figure 4.1 The case X-ray with an arrow pointing to the Boxer's fracture.

with a hand surgeon. Ice, elevation, and analgesia are indicated acutely, particularly in the first 48–72 hours. Initial therapy typically consists of an ulnar gutter splint with the arm in position of function (swelling often prevents optimal casting acutely) extending from below the elbow to the PIP joint (but not including the PIP joint). Fifth metacarpal fractures should be seen by an orthopedic surgeon within 1 week of injury.

Further reading

1 Ashkenaze DM, Ruby LK. Metacarpal fractures and dislocations. *Orthop Clin North Am* 1992;**23**:19–33.
2 Poolman RW, Goslings JC, Lee JB, *et al.* Conservative treatment for closed fifth (small finger) metacarpal neck fractures. *Cochrane Database Syst Rev* 2005;Jul 20 (3):CD003210.

Case 5 | **An elderly man with flank pain**

Answer: C

Diagnosis: Abdominal aortic aneurysm leak

Discussion: Sonographic evaluation of the abdominal aorta requires the real-time visualization of the aorta from the diaphragmatic hiatus to the bifurcation, externally from the xiphoid process to the umbilicus. About 90% of all abdominal

aortic aneurysms (AAAs) are found inferior to the renal arteries, therefore, a normal aorta at or above the renal arteries certainly does not exclude aneurysm. Effective aortic scanning requires differentiation of several retroperitoneal structures. First, identify the vertebral bodies, which are seen as curvilinear hyperechoic structures casting a dense shadow. The aorta lies just anterior and to the left of these. The aorta should not be confused with the inferior vena cava (IVC), which is further to the patient's right compared to the aorta, is thin walled, does not have any branches from its anterior surface, and collapses with deep inspiration and probe pressure. Of note, the IVC, like the aorta, *does* have pulsations. Bowel gas and patient obesity may interfere with the complete real-time visualization of the aorta, resulting in failure to identify a saccular or a localized fusiform AAA. A limited sonographic study mandates alternative imaging if haemodynamically stable. Bedside ultrasound performed by appropriately trained emergency physicians is 95% accurate in measuring the infrarenal aorta.

The aortic diameter is measured from outer wall to outer wall, and is most accurately measured in the transverse plane in the antero-posterior direction. The normal aorta is less than 3 cm in diameter and tapers from diaphragm to its bifurcation. Any dimension greater than this is technically an aneurysm, although problems rarely occur at diameters less than 4 cm. The 5 year rupture rate for aneurysms less than and greater than 5 cm are <4% and >25%, respectively. Many AAAs develop echogenic intraluminal thrombus which can be mistaken for the true aortic walls, as in the present case. Figure 5.1 shows the image from the case with arrows delineating the true extent of the aneurysm. Figure 5.2 shows a lower transverse view than that shown in the case, with the aneurysm and the pseudolumen more readily apparent.

AAAs rupture into the peritoneal cavity only 10–20% of the time. Most of these patients die before reaching the emergency department. More commonly, symptoms are due to acute tears of the vessel wall with varying amounts of acute extravasation. Leaks which are nonlethal tend to occur into the left retroperitoneum. Based on this natural history, the syncope frequently seen in patients with acute AAA is most likely due to pain and ensuing vasovagal response rather than massive hemorrhage. For this reason, it is more useful to speak of "acute" or "symptomatic" rather than "ruptured" AAA. Any aneurysm causing acute symptoms should be treated with equal emergency, regardless of the patient's current vital signs, hemodynamic status, or evidence of hemorrhage. Overall mortality for ruptured AAA is 50%. Early recognition, preparation for potentially rapid and fatal hemodynamic decompensation, emergent surgical consultation, and operative intervention are necessary for optimal management.

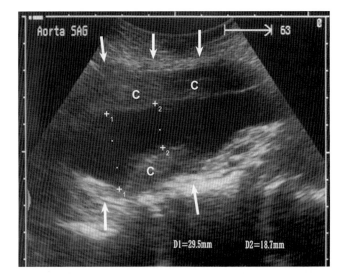

Figure 5.1 Sagittal view of the aorta from the case described with arrows delineating the true extent of the aneurysm (C, clot).

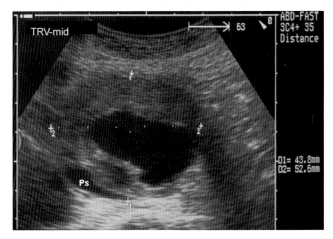

Figure 5.2 A lower transverse view of the aorta than that view shown in Figure 5.1, with the aneurysm and the pseudolumen more readily apparent (Ps, pseudolumen).

Further reading

1 Barkin AZ, Rosen CL. Ultrasound detection of abdominal aortic aneurysm. *Emerg Med Clin North Am* 2004;**22**(3):675–82.
2 Aburahma AF, Woodruff BA, Stuart SP, *et al.* Early diagnosis and survival of ruptured abdominal aortic aneurysms. *Am J Emerg Med* 1991;**9**(2):118–21.

Case 6 | **An immigrant child with skin lesions**

Answer: A

Diagnosis: Coining

Discussion: Often mistaken for abuse, coining is a common practice throughout Asian cultures. Referred to as "cao gio" (scratch the wind) in Vietnamese, this practice is a folk remedy intended to treat fevers, headache, and other maladies by enabling the release of "bad winds" from the body. Coining can mimic physical abuse and is of great concern to many practitioners who do not realize the generally benign nature of this cultural practice. The remedy produces linear micro-ecchymoses as a result of rubbing a coin on oiled skin. These erythematous, striped lesions generally last 1 or 2 weeks but can transit into lasting areas of hyperpigmentation.

Aside from coining, there are many other culturally specific practices that can result in impressive patterned ecchymosis. In cupping for example, cotton is soaked in alcohol and ignited inside a glass cup. Once the glass is heated and oxygen removed, the cotton is withdrawn and the cup placed immediately on the skin, creating a vacuum. This results in circular ecchymotic areas that can also look bizarre and concerning. This remedy is practiced primarily by Russian immigrants as well as in Asian and Mexican-American cultures. Other therapies such as moxibustion can cause small burns, similar to cigarette burns, and also can elicit concern.

Despite the generally benign nature of the aforementioned practices, these and other culturally specific remedies can inadvertently cause harm. Specifically, severe burns can result from cupping and coining. Additionally, salting, another Asian custom, can result in hypernatremia. Uvulectomy, as practiced in several African countries, can lead to infection, as can the small, deep, therapeutic burns known as maquas that are part of a traditional Arabic therapy.

Essential to evaluating these patients is an open-minded, nonjudgmental approach to the history and to patient care. Without having an appreciation for the deep-rooted beliefs of other cultures, the clinician risks alienating his or herself from the patient and family, in turn missing out on potentially vital historical information and ultimately disserving the patient.

Further reading

1 Crutchfield CE, Bisig TJ. Coining. *New Engl J Med* 1995; **332**(23): 1552.
2 Hansen KK. Folk remedies and child abuse: a review with emphasis on caida de mollera and its relationship to shaken baby syndrome. *Child Abuse Negl* 1998;**22**(2): 117–27.
3 Flores G, Rabke-Verani J, Pine W, Sabharwal A. The importance of cultural and linguistic issues in the emergency care of children. *Pediatr Emerg Care* 2002;**18**(4):271–84.

Case 7 | **Wrist pain following a fall**

Answer: C

Diagnosis: Perilunate dislocation

Discussion: Perilunate dislocation usually occurs in the setting of a fall on outstretched hand (FOOSH). Diagnosis is suggested by history of a hyperextension injury with persistent pain, swelling, and deformity; however, patients may present innocuously complaining only of a "sprained wrist." The most common clinical association is median nerve injury, but ulnar nerve injury, arterial injury, and tendon damage may also occur. Many clinicians believe that perilunate injuries are generally under-diagnosed due to their subtle nature, but it is estimated that they comprise <10% of all wrist injuries.

Perilunate injuries can be classified into four stages:

Stage I: Scapholunate dissociation. Characterized by the "Terry Thomas sign," which is widening of the scapholunate joint on the PA radiograph (named after a British comedian with a gap between his front teeth).

Stage II: Perilunate dislocation. The lunate remains in position relative to the distal radius and the capitate is dorsally dislocated. Best seen on the lateral radiograph (left).

Stage III: Perilunate dislocation with dislocation of triquetrium. This is best seen on the PA radiograph (right) with overlap of the triquetrium on the lunate or hamate.

Stage IV: Lunate dislocation. The lunate rotates in a volar direction resulting in a triangular appearance on the PA radiograph. On the lateral radiograph the lunate will look like a cup tipped forward toward the palm which is known as the "spilled teacup sign."

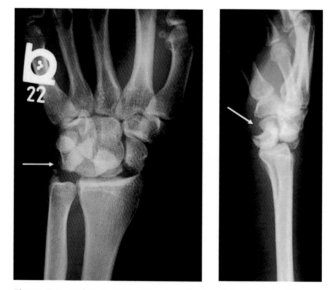

Figure 7.1 Perilunate dislocation (seen best on lateral view) with ulnar styloid fracture (arrow on anteroposterior view).

Perilunate fractures and dislocations require open reduction and internal fixation as soon after the injury as possible. Closed reduction may be attempted in the emergency department until the definitive procedure can be performed.

Further reading

1 Perron AD, Brady WJ, Keats TE, Hersh RE. Orthopedic pitfalls in the ED: lunate and perilunate injuries. *Am J Emerg Med* 2001;**19**(2):157–62.

2 Soejima O, Iida H, Naito M. Transscaphoid–transtriquetral perilunate fracture dislocation: report of a case and review of the literature. *Arch Orthop Trauma Surg* 2003; **123**(6):305–7.

Case 8 | **Rash in a child with epilepsy**

Answer: A

Diagnosis: Toxic epidermal necrolysis (secondary to phenytoin)

Discussion: There are a number of drug hypersensitivity syndromes (DHSs) reported in the literature, including erythema multiforme (EM), Stevens–Johnson syndrome (SJS), and toxic epidermal necrolysis (TEN). These three DHSs represent a spectrum of a disease, rather than distinct clinical entities.

EM is an acute self-limited eruption characterized by a distinctive clinical eruption, the hallmark of which is the target lesion, with variable mucous membrane involvement. The initial lesion is a dull red macule that expands slightly to a maximum of 2 cm within 2 days. In the center, a small papule or vesicle develops, flattens, and then becomes clear. The periphery gradually changes from red and raised to violaceous and forms a typical concentric target lesion.

SJS is an immune-complex-mediated hypersensitivity complex that is a severe expression of EM. SJS typically involves both the skin and the mucous membranes. Significant involvement of oral, nasal, eye, vaginal, urethral, gastrointestinal, and lower respiratory tract mucous membranes may develop in the course of the illness. SJS is a dermatologic emergency with the potential for severe morbidity and death.

TEN is also an acute dermatologic emergency characterized by widespread erythematous macules and target lesions with full-thickness epidermal necrosis and involvement of more than 30% of the cutaneous surface. There is commonly a prodrome where the patient will complain of progressive skin tenderness, fever, malaise, conjunctival irritation, headache, myalgias, nausea, vomiting, and diarrhea. It is not uncommon for health care providers to misdiagnose the rash at the early stage as a simple viral illness. The skin lesions begin as morbilliform, EM-like, with initial tender erythema. Blisters then form and become confluent. The entire thickness of the epidermis becomes necrotic and shears off. A positive Nikolsky's sign is present if, when lateral pressure is put on the skin with the thumb, the epidermis appears to slide over the underlying dermis. Nails may be lost. The scalp, palms, and soles may be less severely involved, but all mucus membranes (lips, buccal, conjunctiva, genital, anal) are affected. Multi-organ involvement may occur, with blindness, respiratory failure, encephalitis, hepatitis, myocarditis, nephritis, and thyroiditis all reported. The mortality rate associated with TEN can approach 40%.

It is important to review the medication list when patients present with a rash. Health care providers commonly confuse

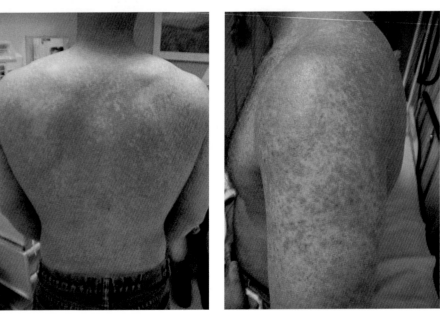

Figure 8.1 A patient with a DHS secondary to sulfa allergy. This case was caught early and his rash resolved shortly after discontinuation of trimethoprim–sulfamethoxazole. If he was misdiagnosed and he continued the causative medication, his condition may have progressed to SJS or TEN.

drug hypersensitivity reactions with "viral exanthems" because there is often preceding fever and malaise.

For all DHSs, prompt withdrawal of the suspected drug(s), good supportive care, and referral to a burn unit in cases of SJS or TEN are the mainstays of therapy. Beyond these simple measures, there is a lack of strong supportive evidence of the benefit of other specific therapies. Most authors reserve antibiotics for proven infections rather than prophylactic administration. Temporary semi-synthetic skin substitute application in areas of denuding has been shown to decrease pain, reduce fluid loss, reduce sepsis, and increase wound healing. Corticosteroids have long been used in the management of SJS or TEN. However, there are multiple studies documenting no demonstrable benefit to steroids for SJS or TEN. Further, there is literature that suggests increased mortality with steroid use.

Further reading

1 Chave TA, Mortimer NJ, Sladden MJ, *et al.* Toxic epidermal necrolysis: current evidence, practical management and future directions. *Br J Dermatol* 2005;**153**:241–53.
2 Letko E, Papaliodis DN, Papaliodis GN, *et al.* Stevens–Johnson syndrome and toxic epidermal necrolysis: a review of the literature. *Ann Allerg Asthma Immunol* 2005;**94**(4):419–36.

Case 9 | **Dark urine in an immigrant**

Answer: B

Diagnosis: Acute hemolysis secondary to glucose-6-phosphate dehydrogenase (G6PD) deficiency and favism

Discussion: G6PD deficiency, the most common human enzymatic disease of red blood cells, is an inherited X-linked disorder with a high prevalence in individuals of African, Middle Eastern, Southern European, Southeast Asian, and Oceanian descent. G6PD is involved in the production of NADPH, which maintains glutathione and other proteins, in the reduced state when erythrocytes are subjected to oxidant stress. Conditions of oxidant stress, including infection, drugs with a high redox potential such as the antimalarial primaquine and sulfa drugs, and favism (broad bean ingestion), produce hemolysis of deficient erythrocytes in susceptible individuals. Favism has also been reported in breast-fed infants of mothers who ate fava beans. Most individuals who are G6PD remain clinically asymptomatic. Sequestration of damaged erythrocytes occurs in the liver and spleen. Symptom severity depends on the number of erythrocytes destroyed. Anemia stimulates erythropoiesis, with an increase in more oxidant-tolerant reticulocytes in 5 days.

Favism results from the presence of two beta-glycosides in fava beans, vicine, and convicine. These are cleaved by intestinal beta-glucosidase to produce the pyrimidine aglycones divicine and isouramil, which reduce the activity of catalase and lower the concentration of reduced glutathione. This, for unclear reasons, does not produce favism every time affected individuals eat broad beans, but the amount eaten and the degree to which the beans are cooked are important factors.

The fall in hemoglobin is acute and often severe, and may be fatal without transfusion. With favism, the spun urine classically shows hemoglobinuria, with 0–1 RBC and a clear red supernatant. The blood smear will show anisocytosis, polychromasia, poikilocytosis, and "blister cells." Serum hemoglobin (3–4 g fall) and haptoglobin will be low, while lactate dehydrogenase and unconjugated bilirubin will be elevated.

In this patient, G6PD testing showed decreased enzyme activity. He responded well to transfusion. He was educated regarding oxidant stressors to avoid.

Further reading

1 Corchia C, Balata A, Meloni GF, Meloni T. Favism in a female newborn infant whose mother ingested fava beans before delivery. *J Pediatr* 1995;**127**:807–8.
2 Galiano S, Gaetani GF, Barabino A, *et al.* Favism in the African type of glucose 6-phosphate dehydrogenase deficiency. *Br Med J* 1990;**300**:236–9.
3 Meloni T, Forteleoni G, Meloni GF. Marked decline of favism after neonatal glucose-6-phosphate dehydrogenase screening and health education: the Northern Sardinian experience. *Acta Haematol* 1992;**87**:29–31.

Case 10 | **Fever and drooling in a child**

Answer: C

Diagnosis: Retropharyngeal abscess

Discussion: Retropharyngeal abscess (RPA) is primarily a disease of childhood, and most frequently occurs in children between ages of 2 and 4 years. Infections are most common in this age group because the retropharyngeal lymph nodes that drain the nasopharynx, middle ear, and posterior paranasal sinuses occupy the prevertebral space. These nodes begin to involute by the age of 5 years. Clinical symptoms of RPA include fever, irritability, neck stiffness/pain (worse with extension), and drooling. In severe cases respiratory distress and stridor may be present as a result of airway compromise. On physical examination, one might see bulging of the posterior pharyngeal wall, although given the age of the involved patients and the likely difficulty of the examination, this may not be obvious. Involved organisms are most commonly group A *Streptococcus, Staphylococcus aureus*, and the anaerobes that occupy the oral cavity.

Radiographic evaluation of children with the above complaints mandates differentiation of RPA from other etiologies including epiglottitis, foreign body aspiration, and meningitis. Lateral neck images are often obtained in an effort to evaluate the width of the prevertebral space and anterior displacement of the airway. To avoid artificially widened spaces, the child's neck should be kept in full extension during inspiration. Pathology should be suspected if the retropharyngeal space is greater than 7 mm at C2 or 14 mm at C6, such as is noted in this case.

Computerized tomography (CT) scanning with contrast is frequently used to further characterize the nature of the swelling and is more sensitive in evaluating the difference between cellulitis and true abscess. Furthermore, CT can help to determine the extension of the infection into neighboring regions and the extent of airway compromise. The management of RPA is appropriate antibiotic coverage with or without surgical drainage. Patients with obvious respiratory distress are the most likely candidates for drainage and CT scan can help to guide the surgical approach. In more subtle cases, CT findings can be useful in determining whether or not surgical drainage is required. Radiologic procedures should only be performed in those who are medically stable, appropriately monitored, and with emergent airway equipment at bedside. The immediate threat to life is loss of the airway followed by overwhelming infection.

Further reading

1 Craig F, Schunk J. Retropharyngeal abscess in children: clinical presentation, utility of imaging and current management. *Pediatrics* 2003;**111**(6):1394–8.

2 Al-Sabah B, Bin Salleen H, Hagr A, *et al*. Retropharyngeal abscess in children: 10-year study. *J Otolaryngol* 2004; **33**(6):352–5.

Case 11 | **Altered mental status with an abnormal electrocardiogram**

Answer: D

Diagnosis: Hyperkalemia

Discussion: The electrocardiogram (ECG) (Figure 11.1) reveals a wide complex rhythm with an irregular rate. Upon review of the medical record, a history of chronic renal failure with hemodialysis was noted; laboratory analysis confirmed the suspicion for hyperkalemia with a serum potassium of 8.3 mEq/dL. With this history and laboratory result, the ECG diagnosis of the wide complex rhythm – with a sine-wave configuration – is sinoventricular rhythm due to hyperkalemia. While the laboratory results do, in fact, confirm the diagnosis, the clinician should consider this diagnostic possibility based upon the initial ECG rhythm.

Hyperkalemia, a common life-threatening metabolic emergency, is most often diagnosed in patients with renal failure. Hyperkalemia may present with lethargy and weakness as

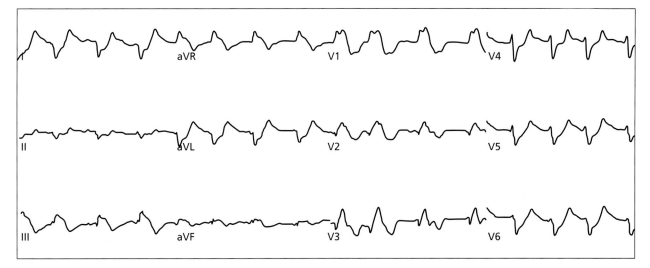

Figure 11.1 Wide QRS complex rhythm with sine-wave configuration.

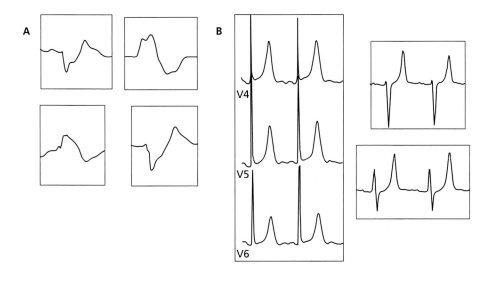

Figure 11.2 A Wide QRS complex sine-wave configuration in pronounced hyperkalemia. **B** Prominent T-waves of hyperkalemia – tall, narrow, peaked, and symmetric.

the sole manifestation; alternatively, the patient may demonstrate significant ECG abnormality in addition to the mental status and constitutional signs. Both ECG morphologic and rhythm findings are seen in these patients; a subset of these patients, those with widening of the QRS complex, are at significant risk of decompensation and death. While serum chemistry analysis is the primary diagnostic investigation, the syndrome is suggested with certain ECG findings, including prominent T-waves and widened QRS complex. In fact, because of the potential delay in laboratory analysis, prompt diagnosis of life-threatening hyperkalemia can be made by the ECG.

From a pathophysiologic perspective, increasing potassium levels are associated with depressed electrical conduction. Furthermore, significant variation is noted with respect to serum potassium levels and clinical manifestation; in general, sudden or rapid increases in the potassium concentration in serum are associated with earlier development of clinical illness, including ECG abnormalities. It is important to note, however, that the relationship between potassium levels and ECG changes may vary between different patients. It is also important to realize that the ECG is not a reliable test for mild to moderate hyperkalemia. Mild levels of hyperkalemia are associated with acceleration of terminal repolarization, resulting in T-wave changes (Figure 11.2B and Table 11.1) – namely an increase in amplitude of the T-wave. The T-wave is described as prominent with descriptors such as "tenting" or "peaking" of the T-wave; the T-wave is tall, narrow, and symmetric. The "peaked" T-wave is generally considered the earliest sign of hyperkalemia. Mild to moderate hyperkalemia causes depression of conduction, resulting in progressive prolongation of the PR and QRS intervals (Figures 11.1 and 11.2A; Table 11.1). The atrial myocardium is particularly sensitive to hyperkalemia. P-wave amplitude lessens with progressive increase in the serum potassium; eventually, the P-wave will disappear, even in the presence of continued sinus node activity, producing the "sinoventricular" rhythm of significant hyperkalemia. With minimal QRS complex

Table 11.1 Electrocardiographic manifestations of serum hyperkalemia relative to serum potassium level

Serum potassium	Electrocardiographic manifestations
5.5–6.5 mEq/L	Prominent T-wave – Tall, narrow, symmetric – Most prominent in precordial leads
6.5–8.0 mEq/L	Decreased P-wave amplitude Prolonged PR interval Prominent T-wave QRS complex widening (minimal to sine-wave configuration) Dysrhythmia – Atrioventricular block – Intraventricular block – Bradycardia – Ventricular ectopy
>8.0 mEq/L	Sinoventricular rhythm – Absence of P-wave – QRS complex widening, progressing to sine-wave QRS complex Ventricular tachycardia Ventricular fibrillation Asystole

widening, the ECG can mimic a bundle branch block appearance. The QRS complex continues to widen and may eventually blend with the T-wave by creating a "sine-wave" appearance (Figures 11.1 and 11.2A). Continued increases in the potassium level eventually produce ventricular fibrillation.

The management of the patient with hyperkalemia includes therapies aimed at the stabilization of the myocardium (calcium), temporary shifting of the excess potassium intracellularly (dextrose, insulin, beta-adrenergic agonists, magnesium, and sodium bicarbonate), and ultimate removal of the potassium from the body (gastrointestinal binding resins and hemodialysis). The goals of therapy are a reduction of the serum potassium level coupled with a stabilization of the myocardial cell membrane. Response to therapy is often prompt with visualization noted on the ECG monitor; caution is advised, however, that improvement is often transient until definitive therapy (i.e. hemodialysis) is provided. The most appropriate initial medication is calcium, delivered in the form of either calcium chloride or calcium gluconate. Calcium works by restoring a more appropriate electrical gradient across the cell membrane. Caution is advised in the setting of hyperkalemia related to digoxin toxicity; anecdotal reports suggest a tendency toward asystole in this clinical setting. Several agents are capable of transiently moving the potassium from the extracellular to intracellular space, including glucose, insulin, beta-adrenergic agonists (i.e. albuterol), magnesium, sodium bicarbonate, and intravenous saline. Ultimate lowering of the serum potassium is accomplished with binding resins (e.g. sodium polystyrene) and/or hemodialysis.

Further reading

1 Amal Mattu A, Brady WJ, Robinson D. Electrocardiographic manifestations of hyperkalemia. *Am J Emerg Med* 2000;**18**:721–9.
2 Schaefer TJ, Wolford RW. Disorders of potassium. *Emerg Med Clin North Am* 2005;**23**(3):723–47.

Case 12 | **Purulent eye discharge in an adult**

Answer: C

Diagnosis: Bacterial conjunctivitis due to *Neisseria gonorrhea*

Discussion: Bacterial conjunctivitis can affect patients of all ages. The causative organisms are numerous and differ in frequency between adults and children. Symptoms of bacterial conjunctivitis include hyperemia, ocular discharge, eyelids matted together in the morning, and foreign body sensation.

Hyperacute, purulent conjunctivitis is the most severe form of bacterial conjunctivitis and is classically associated with *Neisseria gonorrhea*. This infection may progress rapidly to involve the cornea, resulting in scarring or perforation. The abrupt onset of symptoms and hyperpurulent discharge will often bring these patients to the emergency department for evaluation and treatment.

Broad spectrum, topical antibiotic therapy is sufficient for most acute conjunctival infections. However, any suspicion of gonococcal infection requires laboratory evaluation. Gram staining, looking for Gram negative, intracellular diplococci, along with culture and sensitivity of conjunctival scrapings should be done prior to treatment. Cultures should be placed on chocolate agar, blood agar, or Thayer–Martin media.

Treatment for gonococcal conjunctivitis requires topical and systemic therapy. Ceftriaxone, 1 g intravenous or intramuscular, and topical ciprofloxacin ophthalmic drops every 2 hours are usually effective along with irrigation with sterile saline four times a day. Treatment for concomitant chlamydial coinfection and evaluation of patient's sexual partners are also recommended.

Further reading

1 Deschenes J, Seamone C, Baines M. The ocular manifestations of sexually transmitted diseases. *Can J Ophthalmol* 1990; **25**(4):177–85.
2 Harkins T. Sexually transmitted diseases. *Optom Clin* 1994; **3**(4):129–56.

Case 13 | **Wrist pain in a young child**

Answer: E

Diagnosis: Buckle fracture

Discussion: This patient has a buckle fracture (also known as a "Torus" fracture) of the distal radius. A cortical bulge or "buckling" occurring at the metaphysis of a long bone is diagnostic of this type of fracture. Lateral films often show signs of buckling better than on the anterior–posterior view. Both cortical margins are affected, but a discreet fracture line or trabecular disruption is absent. On occasion, radiographic signs of a fracture are not evident on the initial X-ray and a clinical diagnosis must be pursued. A second set of X-rays 2–3 weeks after the trauma should be obtained. It is important to remember that sprains are rare in 9-year-old children and they do not typically complain about 3 days of pain following minor injuries (Figure 13.1).

The etiology of this type of fracture is typically a fall on outstretched arm injury. It is a compression fracture of the long bone typically occurring in children. Because of the

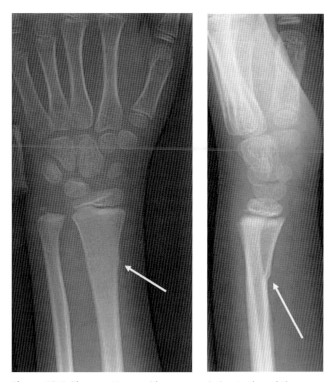

Figure 13.1 The case X-rays with arrows pointing to the subtle buckle fracture.

elasticity of young bones, the dorsal aspect of the cortex is disrupted from the compression injury, while the volar aspect of the cortex is stretched but does not break. The radius is typically solely involved; however, the ulna is not always spared.

The treatment of a buckle fracture has traditionally been managed by placing a well-fitting immobilizing cast for a period of 2–3 weeks. Most see this modality as primarily relieving pain. Some believe that a cast that crosses the elbow is necessary to prevent angulation deformity during healing. However, other authorities have advocated splinting and ace bandages, as these treatments have not demonstrated adverse outcomes. Analgesics, such as ibuprofen, can be administered for pain relief.

Further reading

1 West S, Andrew J, Bebbington A, *et al*. Buckle fractures of the distal radius are safely treated in a soft bandage: a randomized prospective trial of bandage versus plaster cast. *J Pediatr Orthop* 2005;**25**(3):322–5.
2 Symons S, Rowsell M, Bhowal B, Dias JJ. Hospital versus home management of children with buckle fractures of the distal radius: a prospective, randomised trial. *J Bone Joint Surg Brit* 2001;**83**(4):556–60.

Case 14 | **Postprandial abdominal pain**

Answer: D

Diagnosis: Cholelithiasis with evidence of acute cholecystitis

Discussion: The images show a small shadowing gallstone in the gallbladder (GB) neck in Figure 14.1A (triangular arrows) and a large gallstone in the fundus in Figure 14.1B (calipers). The centimeter markers along the top reveal the GB wall (left image, thin straight arrows, and calipers) to be approaching a centimeter in thickness (the upper limit of normal is 3 mm in a non-contracted GB).

The cause of thickened GB walls is non-surgical in more than 50% of cases and is most commonly caused by edema states such as liver disease, renal disease, and congestive heart failure. In these cases, wall thickening is typically uniform throughout the GB, and the wall should maintain its structural integrity, with a characteristic well-defined trilaminar structure of two relatively hyperechoic layers (serosa and mucosa) separated by the thicker hypoechoic muscularis layer. In contrast, the current images show heterogeneous areas of focal edema scattered through the wall (large arrows), with irregular wall thickening and areas of frank mucosal breakdown (short and wide arrows). All these findings are suggestive of an acute

inflammatory process which, combined with the presence of gallstones, is almost certainly acute cholecystitis.

In the ambulatory setting cholecystitis rarely occurs without the presence of gallstones. The most accurate diagnostic study for the detection of gallstones is ultrasound, which, combined with its rapidity, makes this a useful application of clinician-performed bedside sonography. In contrast to the presence or absence of gallstones, sonographic findings of cholecystitis can be relatively subtle. The examiner must also check for the presence of the sonographic murphy sign: tenderness elicited by direct probe pressure on the GB, with absence of tenderness when pressure is applied elsewhere on the abdomen. Nuclear scintigraphy is more accurate in the diagnosis of cholecystitis but can overlook stones causing resolved biliary colic and is not readily available in most emergency departments. Oral cholecystography and endoscopic retrograde cholangiopancreatography (ERCP) are not practical in the emergency department settings.

Several studies have shown that the clinical exam is inaccurate in the identification of biliary colic, and in the differentiation between colic and cholecystitis. While the majority of

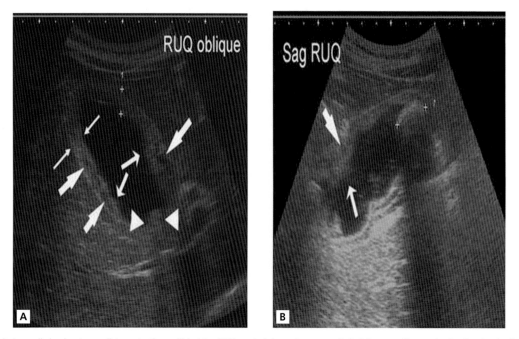

Figure 14.1 **A** A small shadowing gallstone in the gallbladder (GB) neck (triangular arrows). **B** A large gallstone in the fundus (calipers).

patients with biliary disease have some combination of upper abdominal pain, nausea, vomiting, fever, right upper quadrant tenderness, and leukocytosis, many patients with these symptoms do not have biliary disease. Biliary pain is most commonly in the epigastrium (not the right upper quadrant) lasting 5–24 hours (average is 16). Patients most commonly describe biliary pain as "steady" in character, not "colicky". Pain that occurs "in waves" is much more likely to be *non*-biliary in origin. It reaches peak intensity soon after onset, and gradually subsides thereafter. Many patients with proven cholecystitis (based on pathology or nuclear scintigraphy) do not have fever or leukocytosis.

Further reading

1 Shea JA, Berlin JA, Escarce JJ. Revised estimates of diagnostic test sensitivity and specificity in suspected biliary tract disease. *Arch Int Med* 1994;**154**:2573–81.
2 Trowbridge RL, Rutkowski NK, Shojania KG. Does this patient have cholecystitis? *J Am Med Assoc* 2003;**289**(1):80–6.
3 Gruber PJ, Silverman RA, Gottesfeld S. Presence of fever and leukocytosis in acute cholecystitis. *Ann Emerg Med* 1996; **28**(3):273–7.
4 Singer AJ, McCracken G, Henry MC. Correlation among clinical, laboratory, and hepatobiliary scanning findings in patients with acute cholecystitis. *Ann Emerg Med* 1996;**28**(3):267–72.

Case 15 | **An elderly man from a house fire**

Answer: E
Diagnosis: Smoke inhalation with associated burns
Discussion: One of the primary clinical problems in the smoke inhalation victim is respiratory compromise. The patient may have voice changes and his speech may progressively worsen as the airway becomes increasingly edematous. Stridor and acute respiratory arrest may develop rapidly if the patient is not managed appropriately. The patient may have difficulty managing airway secretions with copious quantities of soot containing sputum being expectorated. Visualization of

the vocal cords by direct laryngoscopy may be difficult due to soot accumulation, secretions, or edema. Auscultation of the chest may demonstrate rhonchi, rales, and wheezing suggestive of acute lung injury (ALI). ALI is defined as diffuse alveolar filling of acute onset with hypoxemia but without left atrial hypertension. The most severe manifestation of ALI is the acute respiratory distress syndrome and is defined based on the patient's ability to oxygenate. Bronchospasm may occur, particularly in patients with underlying reactive airway disease. In patients with severe bronchospasm, breath sounds, including wheezing, may be virtually inaudible. Tachycardia and tachypnea may be pronounced, and hypotension may occur with faint or no peripheral pulses noted.

Critical airway compromise may be present upon arrival at the hospital or it may develop soon after arrival. A major pitfall in managing a patient with smoke inhalation is failing to appreciate that rapid deterioration is possible. The history and physical findings help to determine significant smoke exposure and the potential for clinical deterioration. Upper airway patency must be evaluated and rapidly established. When obvious oropharyngeal burns are observed, upper airway injury is almost certain even if overt injuries are not present. Distal airway injury may be present and underestimated. When evidence of upper airway injury exists, early endotracheal intubation should be performed under controlled circumstances. Indications for early intubation include coma, stridor, or full-thickness circumferential neck burns. Other signs suggestive of an increased risk for airway compromise include facial burns, carbonaceous sputum, edema of the posterior pharynx, and singed nasal hairs. Aggressive fluid resuscitation of the burned patient is necessary, but may contribute to upper airway edema. Therefore, early intubation may be necessary in the patient with dermal burns undergoing aggressive fluid management. Treatment of progressive respiratory failure includes mechanical ventilation, continuous positive airway pressure, positive end expiratory pressure, and vigorous clearing of pulmonary secretions. Carbon monoxide poisoning may also be present in the burned patient. It is treated with supplemental oxygen therapy, administered by high flow, tight-fitting mask, endotracheal tube, or hyperbaric oxygen therapy depending on the circumstances.

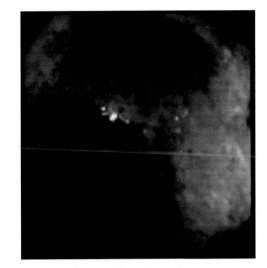

Figure 15.1 Bronchoscopy of the patient in this case. Note the edema of the airways and the black soot deposition on the mucosa.

Further reading

1 Miller K, Chang A. Acute inhalation injury. *Emerg Med Clin North Am* 2003;**21**(2):533–57.
2 Kuo DC, Jerrard DA. Environmental insults: smoke inhalation, submersion, diving, and high altitude. *Emerg Med Clin North Am* 2003;**21**(2):475–97.
3 Lee-Chiong TL. Smoke inhalation injury. *Postgrad Med J* 1999; **105**(2):55–62.

Case 16 | **Back pain following a fall**

Answer: B

Diagnosis: Lumbar wedge fracture

Discussion: Spinal fractures resulting from axial compression form a continuum from minor wedge compression and end plate fractures to severe burst fractures with spinal canal compromise. More than 150,000 persons in North America sustain fractures of the vertebral column each year, and 11,000 of these patients sustain spinal cord injuries. The thoracolumbar spine and lumbar spine are the most common sites for fractures due to the high mobility of the lumbar spine compared to the more rigid thoracic spine.

When the clinician encounters an axial compression injury to the spine, a determination must be made as to whether it is a simple (and stable) wedge fracture versus a more severe injury, such as a burst fracture with potential spinal instability. The most benign injuries, such as end plate fractures or wedge fractures involving a 50% or less loss of vertebral height, are relatively easy to care for and the emphasis is placed on providing the patient with adequate analgesia. Wedge fractures where there is more than 50% loss of height, multiple adjacent wedge fractures, significant kyphotic angulation, or any concern for posterior vertebral involvement or canal compromise are considered high risk.

Radiographically, the clinician should look for certain findings on the lateral radiograph to help make the determination whether an injury represents a wedge fracture versus a burst fracture. Besides the 50% body height cut-off, the clinician needs to examine for posterior cortical disruption of the vertebral body, loss of posterior vertebral height, or a compression angle >20%.

A common question with these injuries is "which patients need advanced imaging in the emergency department" for

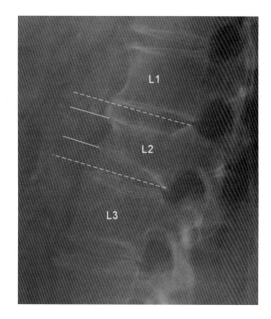

Figure 16.1 Enlarged lateral lumbar spine film of the described patient. The L2 wedge fracture is plainly evident. There is loss of approximately 50% of the original vertebral height (compare dashed lines to solid lines). The posterior vertebral appears to be intact.

clarification of these injuries. Axial imaging (with computed axial tomography or CT) is the gold standard for inspecting the posterior elements of the vertebra, as well as assuring the integrity of the spinal canal. Two studies (Campbell 1995, Ballock 1992) have specifically looked at the clinician's ability to determine wedge versus burst morphology on plain film as opposed to CT. In 17–20% of cases, burst fractures were misinterpreted on the plain films and thought to represent simple wedge injuries.

In summary, while the wedge fracture is a relatively benign condition, the clinician must be sure that it does not, in fact, represent a burst injury with a markedly increased potential for morbidity. In wedge fractures with 50% or greater loss of height, evidence of posterior cortical disruption, or a compression angle >20 degrees, it is wise to utilize CT to determine whether there is more extensive involvement.

Further reading

1 Ballock RT, Mackersie R, Abitol JJ, Cervilla V, Resnick D, Garfin SR. Can burst fractures be predicted from plain radiographs? *J Bone Joint Surg Br* 1992;**74**(1):147–50.
2 Campbell SE, Phillips CD, Dubovsky E, Cail WS, Omary RA. The value of CT in determining potential instability of simple wedge-compression fractures of the lumbar spine. *Am J Neuroradiol* 1995;**16**(7):1385–92.
3 Terregino CA, Ross SE, Lipinski MF, Foreman J, Hughes R. Selective indications for thoracic and lumbar radiography in blunt trauma. *Ann Emerg Med* 1995;**26**(2):126–9.
4 Wintermark M, Mouhsine E, Theumann N, Mordasini P, van Melle G, Leyvraz PF, Schnyder P. Thoracolumbar spine fractures in patients who have sustained severe trauma: depiction with multi-detector row CT. *Radiology* 2003;**227**(3):681–9.

Case 17 | **A bite to the leg in tall grass**

Answer: D

Diagnosis: Crotalid envenomation

Discussion: Thousands of crotalid snakebites occur each year throughout the world. Crotalids may be distinguished from other species by their triangular shaped heads, elliptical shaped pupils, and a single row of subcaudal scales. They also possess infrared heat-sensing pits, thus the name "pit viper", which enable them to locate prey and guide the direction of strike.

The spectrum of clinical presentation ranges from asymptomatic to cardiovascular collapse and death. Bites from Crotalidae species which do not introduce venom ("dry bites") have been estimated to occur in up to 20% of exposures, such as occurred in this case. Skin lesions may appear as distinct puncture marks or as faint scratches. Pain is frequently the initial complaint. When envenomation occurs, swelling usually begins within minutes of the bite. Tissue necrosis may follow cyanosis, and bleb formation may occur over the affected areas. In addition to direct tissue damage, rhabdomyolysis,

nausea, vomiting and diaphoresis may be seen. Three distinct snakebite-induced coagulopathies have been reported: venom-induced thrombocytopenia, fibrinolysis, and disseminated intravascular coagulation. Coagulopathy may be manifest as petechia, gastrointestinal bleeding, epistaxis, hemoptysis, and bleeding from wounds or phlebotomy sites.

Tourniquets, wound incisions, suction, extraction devises, cryotherapy, heat application, electric shock therapy, and wound excision should not be performed. The bite area should be gently cleansed. Circumferential measurement at several points along the affected limb should be started shortly after the patient's arrival and repeated with neurovascular checks at hourly intervals until swelling subsides.

In those cases where envenomation has occurred, hypotension may be seen secondary to fluid loss through third spacing, vomiting, hemorrhage, or vasovagal effects. Crystalloid administration should begin immediately in these patients and prior to antivenom administration. Pain control usually requires

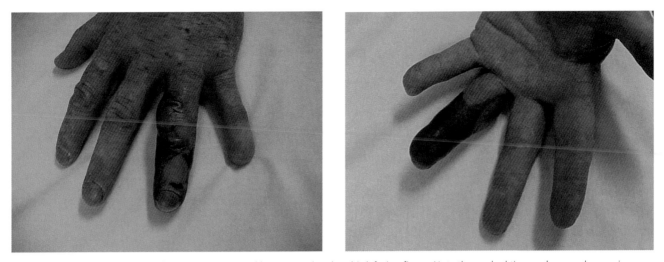

Figure 17.1 A snakebite victim who was envenomated by a copperhead on his left ring finger. Note the marked tissue edema and necrosis that developed around the bite site.

intravenous opioid agents. Prophylactic antibiotics and steroid administration are not recommended.

Currently, two snake antivenoms are approved for treating North American crotaline envenomations: equine derived polyvalent IgG (Wyeth–Ayerst Laboratories) and ovine polyvalent Fab immunoglobulin fragments (CroFab™ from Protherics Inc.). Dosing and mixing of these products are found on the product insert. Pediatric patients should be treated with the same amount of antivenom as adults, regardless of their weight. The most critical decision facing the clinician treating snakebite victims is when antivenom therapy is appropriate. Because anaphylaxis and serum sickness have been associated with the use of antivenom (less commonly with ovine polyvalent Fab), potential risk to the patient must be weighed against benefits. The major indications for antivenom therapy include rapid progression of swelling,

significant coagulation defect, and cardiovascular collapse. Patients who are asymptomatic or have minimal symptoms do not require antivenom.

Patients who remain asymptomatic for 4 hours after the snakebite and who have normal coagulation studies may be released. Symptomatic patients should be considered candidates for hospitalization and the need for antivenom therapy determined.

Further reading

1 Singletary E, Rochman AS, Bodmer JCA, Holstege CP. Envenomations. *Med Clin North Am* 2005;**89**(6):1195–224.
2 Holstege CP, Miller MB, Wermuth M, Furbee B, Curry SC. Crotalid snake envenomation. *Crit Care Clin* 1997;**13**(4):889–921.

Case 18 | **Facial swelling in a patient with poor dentition**

Answer: D
Diagnosis: Submandibular abscess (Ludwig's angina)
Discussion: Infection of the submandibular space occurs when a periapical abscess of the second or third molar penetrates the inner cortex of the mandible and gains access to the area inferior to the insertion of the mylohyoid muscles. As the infection tracks posterior, the sublingual space becomes involved. Ludwig's angina refers to the resultant cellulitis of the submandibular space, beginning in the submaxillary space

and spreading to the sublingual space via the fascial planes. As the submandibular space begins to expand as a result of the cellulitis or abscess, the floor of the mouth becomes indurated and the tongue is forced upward and backward. This can subsequently cause airway obstruction.

Ludwig's angina typically manifests with fever, pain, drooling, trismus, dysphagia, submandibular mass (as visualized in this case), and dyspnea. Airway compromise caused by displacement of the tongue can occur abruptly. Obvious signs of airway obstruction necessitating immediate artificial airway include stridor, dysphonia, and dyspnea. If airway compromise is not imminent and time allows, fiberoptic nasotracheal intubation or tracheostomy, under local anesthesia, should be performed in a multidisciplinary fashion (ideally in the operating room). Some authors recommend early definitive airway intervention even if there are no signs of airway compromise. Abrupt airway closure has occurred in patients with Ludwig's angina despite careful observation. Published reports document that active airway management in the form of endotracheal intubation or tracheotomy was eventually required in 35% of cases of Ludwig's angina. Computerized tomography scans are utilized in select cases to determine the extent of

infection if the patient is medically stable, appropriately monitored, and emergent airway equipment is at bedside. Before antibiotics, nearly half of Ludwig's angina cases died. With broad spectrum antibiotics and prompt surgical care, the mortality rate now is less than 5%.

Further reading

1 Quinn FB. Ludwig angina. *Arch Otolaryngol Head Neck Surg* 1999; **125**(5):599.
2 Saifeldeen K, Evans R. Ludwig's angina. *Emerg Med J* 2004; **21**(2):242–3.
3 Marple BF. Ludwig angina: a review of current airway management. *Arch Otolaryngol Head Neck Surg* 1999;**125**(5):596–9.

Case 19 | **Elbow pain in a child after a fall**

Answer: E

Diagnosis: Fat pad sign

Discussion: The "sail sign" or the "fat pad sign," depicted by the presence of anterior and posterior fat lucencies, is seen on this lateral elbow (Figure 19.1). This sign suggests the potential presence of a supracondylar fracture in children and a radial head or proximal ulna fracture in adults. The anterior fat pad may be seen in a normal radiograph along the anterior, distal humerus, but becomes displaced superior and anterior in the presence of a hemarthrosis from a likely intra-articular fracture. In contrast, the posterior fat pad is not seen in normal radiographs because it lies within the olecranon fossa. The presence of a posterior fat pad is always considered abnormal and a sign of significant distention of the joint capsule from a hemarthrosis. If the posterior fat pad is present in the setting of trauma, there is greater than a 90% incidence of an intra-articular fracture. In the absence of trauma, inflammatory etiologies must be considered, including septic joint, gout, and bursitis.

Another diagnostic technique used to detect less obvious supracondylar fractures is the "anterior humeral line" which involves tracing a line along the anterior surface of the distal humerus through the capitellum. The capitellum should then be divided into three equal sections horizontally. The anterior humeral line should pass through the middle section of the capitellum. If this line transects the anterior rather than the middle section or passes completely anterior to the capitellum, there is likely a supracondylar fracture or physis disruption of the capitellum.

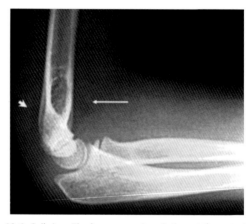

Figure 19.1 Sail sign. The long arrow is pointing at the anterior sail sign; the short arrow is pointing at the posterior sail sign.

The radiocapitellar line is helpful for determining a radial head dislocation or a radial neck fracture. This involves drawing a line through the central portion of the radius. The axis of this line should intersect the capitellum. If the line does not intersect the capitellum, there is likely a dislocation of the radial head or a fracture of the radial neck.

Further reading

1 Goswami G. The fat pad sign. *Radiology* 2002;**222**(2): 419–20.
2 Skaggs DL, Mirzayan R. The posterior fat pad sign in association with occult fracture of the elbow in children. *J Bone Joint Surg Am* 1999;**81**(10):1429–33.

Case 20 | **A man with diffuse facial edema**

Answer: D

Diagnosis: Superior vena cava syndrome

Discussion: The superior vena cava (SVC) is the major conduit for venous blood return from the head, neck, upper extremities, and upper thorax. Obstruction of this blood flow (i.e., compression, infiltration, and thrombosis) results in SVC syndrome (SVCS), which is associated with elevated venous pressure in those structures drained by the SVC. Early signs include periorbital edema and facial swelling that is more prominent in the morning upon awaking. Later signs include thoracic and neck vein distension, plethora of the face, as well as edema and cyanosis of the face and upper extremities. Headache, dyspnea, orthopnea, and cough are also common complaints.

The azygos system of veins receives venous blood from the posterior intercostal veins and therefore drains blood from the chest wall (and esophagus). The azygos veins originate at abdominal levels where they establish important anastomoses with the inferior vena cava (IVC). Obstruction of the SVC above the level of azygos vein allows blood to bypass the SVC obstruction through chest wall collaterals and re-enter the SVC through the azygos venous system. In contrast, when the SVC is obstructed below the level of the azygos vein, blood must travel through the chest wall collateral veins to enter the azygos venous system and subsequently must continue to flow through the azygos system to empty into the IVC. The longer and more convoluted course retards venous return and accounts for the development of more prominent symptoms. Additionally, the severity of symptoms is related to the rate at which the SVC obstruction occurs; the slower the onset of obstruction, the more time for collateral blood flow to develop and the less severe the symptoms.

Historically, SVCS was frequently associated with complications of syphilis and tuberculosis. Today, compression of the SVC by malignant mediastinal tumors accounts for approximately 90% of cases. The most common mediastinal tumors associated with SVCS are bronchogenic carcinoma (70%) and non-Hodgkin's lymphomas (10–15%). The most common histological diagnosis is small cell lung carcinoma. Thrombosis of the SVC is a potential cause of SVCS in patients with a history of intravenous drug abuse and central venous catheter placement.

Immediate management in the emergency department is aimed at alleviating patient symptoms and determining airway patency. Treatment options include supplemental oxygen, elevation of the patient's head, steroids, and diuretics. Depending on the etiology, both radiation therapy and chemotherapy are utilized as primary treatment options for long-term management of SVC compression due to tumors.

Prognosis of patients treated for SVCS is dependent upon the underlying etiology. Histological diagnosis is essential as patients with SVCS resulting from bronchogenic carcinoma have a worse prognosis when compared with lymphoma patients. Overall survival is estimated at 25% at 1 year and 10% at 30 months. The prognosis for SVCS not associated with malignancy is excellent; infectious or thrombotic causes respond to appropriate antibiotics or anticoagulation, respectively.

Further reading

1 Baker GL, Barnes HJ. Superior vena cava syndrome: etiology, diagnosis, and treatment. *Am J Crit Care* 1992;**1**(1):54–64.
2 Wudel LJ, Nesbitt JC. Superior vena cava syndrome. *Curr Treat Options Oncol* 2001;**2**(1):77–91.

Case 21 | **Chest pain and hypotension in an adult male patient**

Answer: B

Diagnosis: Inferoposterior RV AMI

Discussion: The electrocardiogram (ECG) of the case (see page 14) reveals sinus bradycardia at approximately 50 beats/minute with ST segment elevation in leads III and aVf consistent with inferior wall ST-elevation myocardial infarction (STEMI); additionally, ST segment depression is seen in leads V1–V3, consistent with either posterior wall acute myocardial infarction (AMI) or anterior wall ischemia; posterior ECG leads V8 and V9 (Figure 21.1A(iii)) demonstrated ST segment elevation, confirming posterior wall AMI. Lastly, ST segment depression with T-wave inversion (case ECG) is noted in leads I and AVL, consistent with reciprocal change.

Posterior wall myocardial infarction refers to AMI of the posterior wall of the left ventricle. This region of the heart is usually perfused by branches of the right coronary artery (prominent posterolateral or posterior descending arteries) or the left circumflex artery. As such, the 12-lead ECG will usually demonstrate an inferior or lateral wall STEMI as well as ST segment depression, prominent R wave, and upright T-wave in the right precordial leads (Figure 21.1A(i) and (ii)). Myocardial infarction involving the posterior wall usually occurs in conjunction with inferior or lateral AMIs; isolated posterior wall myocardial infarction, however, is encountered even less frequently.

The use of posterior ECG leads is more helpful in the evaluation of posterior wall AMI when compared to the standard

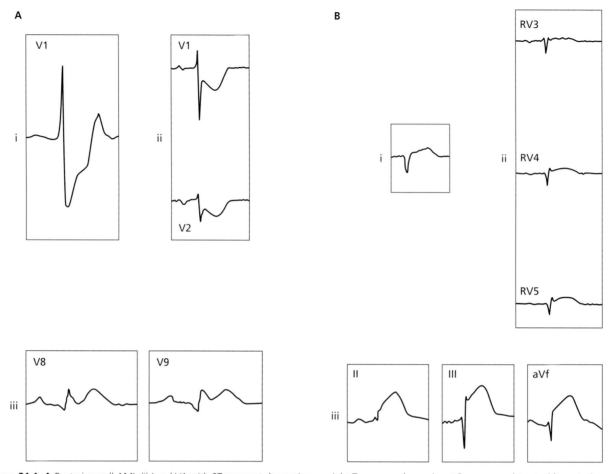

Figure 21.1 A Posterior wall AMI. (i) Lead V1 with ST segment depression, upright T wave, and prominent R wave consistent with posterior wall AMI. (ii) Leads V1 and V2 with ST segment depression and upright T wave, consistent with posterior wall AMI. (iii) Posterior leads V8 and V9 with ST segment elevation, consistent with posterior wall AMI. **B** Right ventricular AMI. (i) Minimal ST segment elevation in lead V1 as seen in RV AMI. (ii) Minimal ST segment elevation in leads RV3–RV5 as seen in RV AMI. (iii) Inferior leads II, III, and aVf in a patient with inferior wall AMI with RV infarction; note the relatively greater magnitude of ST segment elevation in lead III compared to the other inferior leads. This relative imbalance of lead III ST segment elevation results from the axis of imaging of lead III, which most closely observes the right ventricle.

12-lead ECG. ST segment elevation greater than 1 mm in leads V8 and V9 confirms the diagnosis of posterior myocardial infarction (Figure 21.1A(iii)). In fact, the presence of ST segment elevation in the posterior ECG leads is more indicative of posterior AMI than the findings observed in leads V1–V3. The sensitivity of the posterior ECG leads may be as high as 90% for identifying posterior AMI. The magnitude of ST segment elevation is less pronounced in the posterior ECG leads – the posterior leads are located distant from the myocardium, allowing for more resistance to current flow and less pronounced ST segment elevation.

Right ventricular myocardial infarction presents with hypotension, elevated jugular venous pressure, and clear lung fields; the ECG demonstrates ST segment elevation in the inferior (case ECG) and right ventricular leads (Figures 21.1B(i) and (ii)). Right ventricular myocardial infarction occurs in approximately one-third of inferior wall AMIs. The

12-lead ECG reveals ST segment elevation in the inferior leads with the greatest magnitude of elevation in lead III compared to the other leads (Figure 21.1B(iii)); furthermore, lead V1 may also demonstrate ST segment elevation in that this lead (Figure 21.1B(i)), of all the standard leads, most closely images the right ventricle. The use of additional leads greatly increases the ability to diagnose right ventricular infarction.

The addition of lead RV4 provides objective evidence of RV involvement – more so than that noted on the 12-lead ECG. RV infarction is diagnosed with 80–100% sensitivity by ST segment elevation greater than 1 mm in lead RV4. Alternatively, the clinician can use an entire reversal of the precordial leads, namely RV1–RV6 (Figure 21.1B(ii)); in a comparison to the use of single lead RV4, the entire array did not increase the diagnostic ability of the additional lead approach. As with the posterior leads, the magnitude of the ST segment elevation is less pronounced than is usually seen in the standard 12-leads of the ECG; this relatively less pronounced magnitude results from the fact that the right ventricle is composed of considerably less muscle when compared to the left ventricle.

Further reading

1 Zalenski RG, Rydman RJ, Sloan EP, *et al.* Value of posterior and right ventricular leads in comparison to the standard 12-lead electrocardiogram in evaluation of ST-segment elevation in suspected acute myocardial infarction. *Am J Cardiol* 1997;**79**: 1585–97.
2 Brady WJ, Hwang V, Sullivan R, *et al.* A comparison of 12- and 15-lead ECGs in ED chest pain patients: impact on diagnosis, therapy, and disposition. *Am J Emerg Med* 2000;**18**:239–43.
3 Haji SA, Movahed A. Right ventricular infarction – diagnosis and treatment. *Clin Cardiol* 2000;**23**:473–82.

Case 22 | Eye pain after tree branch strike

Answer: B
Diagnosis: Corneal abrasion
Discussion: The photographs on page 15 demonstrate a corneal epithelium defect before and after staining with fluorescein. Patients with corneal abrasions usually complain of sharp pain, foreign body sensation, and tearing. A history of antecedent trauma can usually be elicited. Patients without a history of trauma may be suffering from recurrent corneal erosion syndrome; however, herpes simplex keratitis must also be ruled out in these cases.

Slit lamp examination is critical in the workup of corneal abrasions to determine the size, depth, and location of the abrasion. This also allows the clinician to rule out an anterior chamber reaction and infiltrate indicating a true corneal ulcer. Finally, a careful slit lamp exam with eyelid eversion is necessary to determine the presence of a laceration, penetrating trauma, or foreign body.

Treatment for corneal abrasions should include a topical antibiotic. Erythromycin ointment or trimethoprim/ polymyxin B drops given four times a day are usually sufficient. Contact lens wearers should be given an antibiotic with pseudomonal coverage such as tobramycin or ciprofloxacin. Steroid use should be avoided. Cycloplegic agents such as cyclopentolate or homatropine may be given twice a day for comfort from traumatic iritis. Tetanus immunization status should be assessed and a booster immunization given if necessary. Contact lens wearers must discontinue lens wear until the abrasion has been completely healed for a week.

The primary indication for patching is patient comfort by immobilizing the eyelid from rubbing up and down over the denuded surface. Small or superficial abrasions do not require patching. Larger abrasions may be patched if it makes the patient more comfortable. Abrasions involving vegetative matter or abrasions (or 'those') in contact lens wearers should not be patched. Patients should be reevaluated in 24 hours.

Further reading

1 Shields SR. Managing eye disease in primary care. How to recognize and treat common eye problems. *Postgrad Med* 2000;**108**(5):83–86, 91–6.
2 Mukherjee P, Sivakumar A. Tetanus prophylaxis in superficial corneal abrasions. *Emerg Med J* 2003;**20**(1):62–4.

Case 23 | A missing button battery

Answer: E
Diagnosis: Button battery ingestion with esophageal impaction
Discussion: Ingestions of foreign bodies by toddlers are a relatively common presenting complaint in pediatric emergency departments. Button battery ingestions are managed differently from other foreign body ingestions, such as coin ingestions. Most (about 90%) button battery ingestions are asymptomatic and are based on parental history. Button batteries can cause mucosal injury by leaking battery contents, through electrical discharge, and from pressure necrosis.

Symptoms are not a reliable predictor of the presence of a button battery retained in the gastrointestinal (GI) tract. Radiographic localization of the battery is an important first

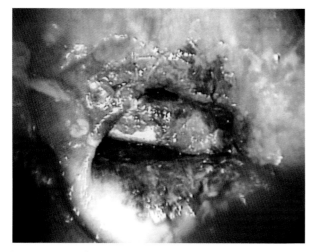

Figure 23.1 Disc battery impaction site as seen through endoscopy.

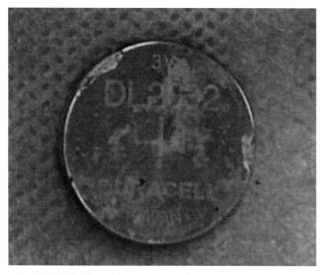

Figure 23.2 The button battery removed.

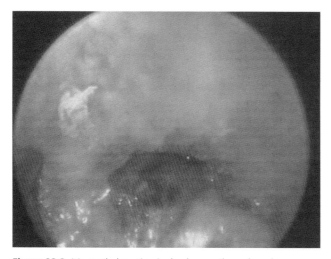

Figure 23.3 Mucosal ulceration is clearly seen through endoscopy following disc battery removal.

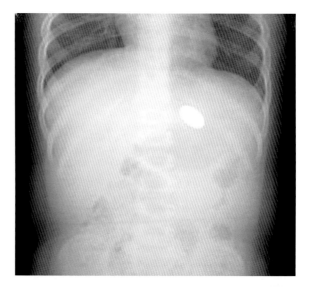

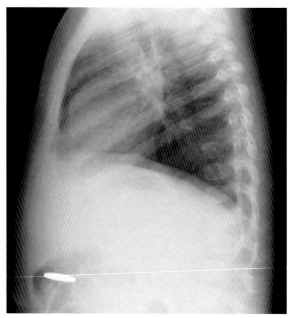

Figure 23.4 Radiographs of an ingested coin. Note both sides are uniformly the same size and the object is thin. Button batteries of similar diameter to a coin are thicker and have a step off; the anode side has a smaller diameter than the cathode side.

step in determining the management strategy, as batteries retained within the esophagus are managed differently from batteries found further along the GI tract. Anteroposterior and lateral films are required to evaluate for an esophageal battery.

Button batteries have an anode and a cathode. This often gives them the characteristic double density shadow caused by the step off between the anode and the cathode. This finding can help to differentiate the battery from an ingested coin (Figure 23.4).

Batteries retained within the esophagus are typically entrapped at one of three levels of anatomic narrowing: the level of the cricopharyngeus muscle, the level of the aortic arch, and the level of the lower esophageal sphincter. Mucosal damage may develop less than 4 hours following ingestion with retention of a button battery within the esophagus. If a button battery is retained in the esophagus, then ulceration, perforation, tracheoesophageal fistula, and esophageal stricture may occur (see Figures 23.1–23.3). However, greater than 90% of all batteries ingested pass through the GI tract without development of complications. As a result of the typically benign course of battery ingestions, it is recommended that batteries distal to the esophagus be followed with outpatient serial abdominal X-rays and stool examination to prove passage. Batteries retained within the esophagus are more likely to have associated complications and should be removed emergently under direct visualization.

Further reading

1 Yardeni D, Yardeni H, Coran AG, Golladay ES. Severe esophageal damage due to button battery ingestion: can it be prevented? *Pediatr Surg Int* 2004;**20**(7):496–501.
2 Samad L, Ali M, Ramzi H. Button battery ingestion: hazards of esophageal impaction. *J Pediatr Surg* 1999;**34**(10): 1527–31.
3 Maves MD, Lloyd TB, Carithers JS. Radiographic identification of ingested disc batteries. *Pediatr Radiol* 1986;**16**(2):154–6.

Case 24 | Acute abdominal pain in pregnancy

Answer: D
Diagnosis: Ruptured ectopic pregnancy
Discussion: In evaluating first trimester pain and bleeding, since no clinical sign or symptom is sufficiently accurate to exclude ectopic, all patients need pelvic ultrasonography. The quantitative beta-HCG level should never be used as a basis for determining the need for ultrasound. In fact, a beta-HCG <1000 mIU/mL has been shown to put a patient with first trimester pain or bleeding presenting to the emergency department at a 4-fold increased risk of ectopic compared with patients whose beta-HCG is >1000 mIU/mL.

The primary focus of the emergency physician performing pelvic ultrasonography for first trimester pain or bleeding is the identification of an intrauterine pregnancy (IUP) to effectively rule out ectopic pregnancy (barring clinical conditions that increase the risk of heterotopic pregnancy, especially use of progestational agents and/or *in vitro* fertilization). The first step is the correct identification of the uterus (see Figure 24.1, arrows), which in this view might be mistaken to include the large retrouterine mass, which is probably clotted blood (arrow heads), and free fluid (FF). The calipers indicate a small intrauterine collection of fluid (dark region) surrounded by a single layer of endometrium (relatively hyperechoic, i.e. whiter on the image).

The earliest sign of IUP is a double decidual sac (DDS, also known as the "double decidual sign"), comprised of two layers of endometrium surrounding an anechoic sac. This sac usually has smooth walls, is eccentrically located, and is rounded in shape (see Figure 24.2), unlike the image of the present case, which shows a single layer of endometrium with a centrally located fluid collection with a "pointy" shape. As can be seen in Figure 24.2, the two layers of the DDS are relatively hyperechoic (white) compared to the surrounding myometrium. Characteristically the outer layer (arrows) usually does not

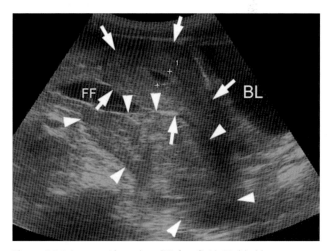

Figure 24.1 Image with markers (FF: free fluid; BL: bladder; see text for details).

form a complete ring around the inner layer (arrow heads). The double decidual sign is used by some as definitive evidence of IUP but considered by others to be too subject to the interpretation of the sonographer to be used to rule out ectopic. If this more conservative approach is taken, the earliest definitive sign of IUP is a yolk sac, followed by a fetal pole and/or intrauterine fetal heart tones.

In the present case, the intrauterine findings would never be sufficient to rule in IUP, regardless of the quantitative beta-HCG. If the patient had not had the large adnexal mass and fluid collection and a beta-HCG <1500 mIU/mL the ultrasound image would have been interpreted as "possible early IUP (viable or non-viable), cannot rule out ectopic." This, assuming the patient is clinically stable and reliable, would allow for discharge with strict instructions to return for repeat evaluation with quantitative beta-HCG assessment in 2–3

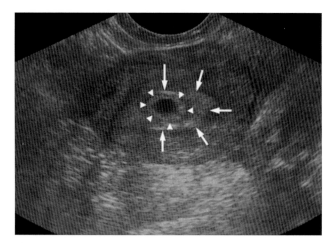

Figure 24.2 Double decidual sac: transverse view of the uterus.

days. This strategy allows for serial quantitative beta-HCG evaluations. If the patient does indeed have a viable early IUP, the beta-HCG will double every 2–3 days. If the beta-HCG falls by half every 2–3 days, the patient most likely has an

intrauterine fetal demise, with abortion either complete or inevitable. She will be followed as an out-patient until her beta-HCG falls to zero. If the beta-HCG does not follow either of these courses, the presence of ectopic is more likely, although abnormal IUP is still a possibility. Gynecological management with continued serial observation, laparoscopy, or dilation and curettage will be determined by clinical factors in combination with patient and physician preference.

With the large adnexal mass seen in the current case, the diagnosis is presumptive ruptured ectopic, regardless of the patient's beta-HCG and clinical appearance. This mandates urgent obstetrical evaluation in the emergency department, with preparations made for the patient to be taken to surgery.

Further reading

1 Reardon RF, Martel ML. First trimester pregnancy. In: *Emergency Ultrasound*. Ma OJ and Mateer JR, Eds. New York: McGraw-Hill, 2003:239–76.
2 Kaplan BC, Dart RG, Varaklis K. Predictive value of history and physical examination in patients with suspected ectopic pregnancy. *Ann Emerg Med* 1999;**33**(3): 283–90.

Case 25 | **Painless penile ulcer**

Answer: D

Diagnosis: Chancre of primary syphilis

Discussion: Genital ulcers occur in sexually active individuals throughout the world. Physicians encountering patients with ulcers tend to rely heavily on history and physical exams in order to make a diagnosis, but this approach may be inappropriate. There is considerable variation and overlap in presentation, and generally additional diagnostic tests need to be performed. Also, concomitant infection with HIV can subtly alter the clinical presentation and compound the difficulty in diagnosing the cause of genital ulcers. Physicians need to use the opportunity of having the patient physically present to administer appropriate therapy under the assumption that follow-up of patients, although ideal, may not occur.

The Centers for Disease Control and Prevention (CDC) currently recommend an approach to the diagnosis and treatment of genital ulcers that relies heavily on clinical presentation and the knowledge of local epidemiological data on the prevalence of causes of genital ulcers in a specific geographic area. In the United States, the three most common causes of genital ulcers in sexually active young adults are herpes simplex virus (HSV), syphilis, and chancroid. The typical clinical presentation of syphilis is a single painless, indurated ulcer with firm, nontender inguinal adenopathy. HSV tends to present with multiple vesicles or a cluster of

painful ulcers preceded by vesiculopustular lesions. Tender inguinal lymph nodes are commonly associated. Chancroid ulcers tend to be multiple, painful, and purulent and are often associated with inguinal lymphadenopathy with fluctuance or overlying erythema. The lymphadenopathy is often unilateral and painful. Lymphogranuloma venereum (LGV) and Granuloma Inguinale rarely cause genital ulcers in the United States.

Diagnostic tests should be performed whenever possible and should be directed toward ascertaining the cause of the genital ulcer as well as screening for commonly occurring coinfections with other sexually transmitted diseases (such as *Chlamydia trachomatis*, *Neisseria gonorrheae*, HIV, hepatitis B, and hepatitis C). For syphilis, options to assist in making a correct diagnosis include serologic tests (i.e. VDRL and RPR), darkfield microscopy and tissue biopsy. For HSV one can do tzank smears, direct fluorescence antibody tests, viral cultures, or polymerase chain reaction (PCR). In the case of *H. ducreyi* (chancroid), Gram stain and culture on selective media are suggested.

Treatment should ideally be directed toward the identified cause. Since diagnostic tests are often not available at the time of presentation or may not always yield a specific cause, or if patient compliance is in question, empiric therapy should be based on the clinical presentation and the epidemiology of the etiologic agents in a given area. If necessary, patients may require treatment for HSV, syphilis, and chancroid (in areas of high incidence) on the day of their initial visit. Also, all patients should be offered HIV counseling and testing on the day of presentation, and they should be counseled about safe-sex practices. Follow-up should be encouraged to discuss laboratory results, ensure treatment was appropriate, and ascertain if healing of the ulcer has occurred. Lastly, patients should be advised to encourage their partners to seek care for potential coexistent sexually transmitted disease.

Further reading

1 Mertz KJ, Tress D, Levine WC, *et al*. Etiology of genital ulcers and prevalence of human immunodeficiency virus coinfection in 10 US cities: the Genital Ulcer Disease Surveillance Group. *J Infect Dis* 1998;**178**(6):1795–8.

2 Morse SA, Trees DL, Htun Y, *et al*. Comparison of clinical diagnosis and standard laboratory and molecular methods for the diagnosis of genital ulcer disease in Lesotho: association with human immunodeficiency virus infection. *J Infect Dis* 1997;**175**(3):583–9.

3 Lynn WA, Lightman S. Syphilis and HIV: a dangerous combination. *Lancet Infect Dis* 2004;**4**(7):456–66.

Case 26 | **Low back pain in car accident victim**

Answer: B

Diagnosis: Anterior teardrop fracture at L5

Discussion: Teardrop fractures result from extensive flexion and compression forces. Common mechanisms producing these forces are seen in motor vehicle crashes, sports injuries, diving accidents, and falls. Teardrop fractures are usually seen in the cervical spine, especially at C2 or C5/C6. They can occur at any level, however, and forced flexion/compression at the waist can cause a lumbar teardrop fracture (see arrow in Figure 26.1 pertaining to X-ray of case above).

All teardrop fractures should be treated as unstable regardless of where they occur. Instability results because there is often complete disruption of ligamentous and bony elements. The anteroinferior fracture segment remains attached to the anterior longitudinal ligament with retropulsion of the vertebral body into the spinal canal. Patients with this type of injury will often present with neurological deficits secondary to cord impingement. Paraplegia, loss of pain, touch, and temperature sensation are common findings.

All trauma patients complaining of back pain or distracting injuries should receive prompt spine radiographs. Teardrop fractures are best seen on a standard lateral view of the spine. Fracture lines are typically seen along the anteroinferior border of the vertebral body, and prevertebral swelling of the soft tissues at the level of trauma combined with subluxation or dislocation of the interfacetal joints characterize this injury. The posterior ligament complex, the posterior longitudinal ligament, the anterior longitudinal ligament, and the intervertebral disk are all disrupted. Severe kyphosis at the injury site can lead to extensive cord damage.

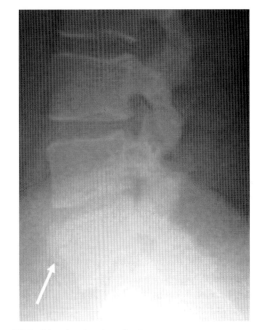

Figure 26.1 A lumbar teardrop fracture.

Patients with radiographic and clinical evidence of a teardrop fracture should remain immobilized in spine precautions and be urgently evaluated by a spinal cord injury team.

Further reading

1 Woolard A, Oussedik S. Injuries to the lumbar spine: identification and management. *Hosp Med* 2005;**66**(7): 384–8.

2 Savitsky E, Votey S. Emergency department approach to acute thoracolumbar spine injury. *J Emerg Med* 1997;**15**(1):49–60.

Case 27 | A gardener with a non-healing rash

Answer: D

Diagnosis: Sporotrichosis

Discussion: Classically known as rose gardener's disease, sporotrichosis is caused by *Sporothrix schenckii*, a dimorphic fungus that is indigenous to many parts of the world. Although this yeast can cause systemic illness (generally in the immune-suppressed host), it most commonly causes localized lymphocutaneous disease. This organism preferentially grows in moss, hay, and soil, and therefore has a predilection for affecting gardeners, farmers, and those sustaining soil contaminated trauma or animal bite wounds.

Lymphocutaneous disease, the most common manifestation of *S. schenckii* exposure, occurs after a precipitating traumatic inoculation of the fungal spores. A papular primary lesion follows, developing weeks to months later. These lesions often become nodular and eventually can ulcerate. With ongoing infection new lesions continue to develop, advancing along the lymphatics proximal to the site of initial inoculation. Occasionally, however, patients will develop only a solitary, plaque-like lesion that usually does not ulcerate. Infection can mimic that of some species of *Mycobacteria* as well as *Leishmaniasis*, *Nocardia*, and *Tularemia*. The vast majority of cases involving *S. schenckii* are lymphocutaneous; however, systemic illness (pulmonary and disseminated disease) does occur after inhalation of *S. schenckii* conidia.

Definitive diagnosis of sporotrichosis can be made by aspirating some of the non-grossly purulent fluid from the individual lesions. Itraconazole is the drug of choice for combating lymphocutaneous disease, with amphotericin B being the therapy of choice for disseminated disease.

Further reading

1 Kauffman CA. Sporotrichosis. *Clin Infect Dis* 1999; **29**(2): 231–6.
2 Kauffman CA, Hajjeh R, Chapman SW. Practice guidelines for the management of patients with sporotrichosis. For the Mycoses Study Group. Infectious Diseases Society of America. *Clin Infect Dis* 2000;**30**(4):684–7.

Case 28 | An immigrant with neck swelling

Answer: D

Diagnosis: Tuberculosis adenitis

Discussion: Tuberculosis (TB), an infection caused by bacilli of the *Mycobacterium tuberculosis* complex (*M. tuberculosis*, *M. bovis*, *M. africanum*, and *M. microti*), usually involves the lungs and causes more deaths worldwide than any other infectious disease. Infection is typically caused by inhalation of infected aerosolized respiratory droplet nuclei from an individual with active pulmonary TB and deposition of these droplets in the terminal alveoli. It has been estimated that one-third of the world's population harbors this infection. Each year TB claims an estimated 3 million lives, the vast majority of which occur in developing countries. TB saw a global resurgence in the 1990s, attributed largely to the HIV epidemic, although inadequate control programs, immigration from developing countries, and other social changes are also important factors. TB was declared a global health emergency in 1993 by the WHO.

The clinical manifestations of TB can be quite varied and may reflect involvement of any system or organ. In immune-competent hosts, a vigorous granulomatous response usually succeeds in stopping progression of infection. In 10–20% of individuals, infection results in clinical disease as a primary infection or after reactivation later in life. Five percent of immuno-competent patients progress to active TB within 2 years of infection, and another 5% do so during the remainder of their lives. The likelihood of progression is increased 2–3-fold in persons with minor immuno-compromise. In significantly immuno-compromised individuals with HIV, progression to disease can occur within 3 months in one-third of patients. In most individuals, the lung serves as both the primary site of infection and also the site of disease manifestation.

Extrapulmonary TB was seen in approximately 15% of patients in the United States before HIV. Extrapulmonary TB, alone or co-existent with pulmonary TB, affects up to two-thirds of HIV patients. Extrapulmonary TB is also more common at the extremes of age and in immigrants from developing countries. Tuberculosis adenitis is the most common form of extrapulmonary TB, occurring in more than 40% of those with extrapulmonary involvement. In developed countries, most cases of lymphadenitis occur in the second and third decade of life. More than 90% of palpable tuberculous lymph nodes occur in the head and neck area. Commonly, several nodes within a chain are involved, with bilateral involvement not uncommon. Generalized lymphadenopathy and hepatosplenomegaly are uncommon. Involvement usually is painless and slowly grows over weeks to months. Most untreated individuals will develop a chronically draining sinus tract. Systemic symptoms, if present, are usually not prominent.

The definitive diagnosis of lymphadenitis requires isolation of the TB in culture. Fine needle aspiration is the diagnostic modality of choice, as incisional biopsies can lead to sinus tract formation. Histopathology shows epithelioid cell granuloma with or without giant cells and caseation necrosis. MTB may be seen within the granuloma, but is often rare. The treatment of choice is 2 months of intensive chemotherapy with daily isoniazid (INH), rifampin (RIF), and pyrazinamide (PZA), supplemented with ethambutol (EMB) or streptomycin (STM) if the prevalence of INH resistance in the community is 4% or higher. If the organisms are susceptible, INH and RIF are continued three times weekly for an additional 4 months.

Further reading

1 Anonymous. Control of tuberculosis in the United States. Joint Statement of the American Thoracic Society, the Centers for Disease Control, and the Infectious Disease Society of America. *Respir Care* 1993;**38**(8):929–39.
2 Ferrer R. Lymphadenopathy: differential diagnosis and evaluation. *Am Fam Physician* 1998;**58**(6):1313–20.
3 Anonymous. Update: adverse event data and revised American Thoracic Society/CDC recommendations against the use of rifampin and pyrazinamide for treatment of latent tuberculosis infection – United States, 2003. *Morb Mortal Wkly Rep* 2003;**52**(31):735–9.
4 Schneider E, Castro KG. Epidemiology of tuberculosis in the United States. *Clin Chest Med* 2005;**26**(2):183–95.

Case 29 | **Fall on an outstretched hand in a young adolescent**

Answer: B

Diagnosis: Distal radius fracture, Salter–Harris type I

Discussion: Musculoskeletal injuries are a common cause for pediatric emergency department (ED) visits. One type of injury involves fracture to the physeal plate (also known as the physis or growth plate) of the growing skeleton. The primary function of the physis is longitudinal bone growth, where bone cells are laid down and subsequently ossified. The nutrient blood supply for this zone of bone growth comes from the epiphysis (the distal or end portion of the bone); normal growth is dependant on an intact vascular pathway. In skeletally immature children, the ligamentous structures will have more relative strength than bone. This relative imbalance in strength means that with trauma, the physis is more likely to suffer a disruptive injury than the adjacent strong, flexible ligament. The Salter–Harris classification system is most commonly used to describe these injuries, which are graded I–V based on the extent of involvement of the physis, epiphysis, and metaphysis. In general, the higher the grade

assigned, the greater the chance of injury to the vascular supply to the physis and subsequent growth abnormalities (Figure 29.1).

The classic patterns described by Salter and Harris are depicted in this case. Type I fractures are seen most frequently in infants and toddlers, representing approximately 5% of physeal injuries. The epiphysis separates from the metaphysis; in fact, there is no osseous fracture to the epiphysis or metaphysis. Salter–Harris type II injuries are the most common type encountered, accounting for 75% of physeal injuries. The line of fracture runs through the hypertrophic cell zone of the physis and then out through a segment of metaphyseal bone. Salter–Harris type III injury is an intra-articular fracture of the epiphysis with extension through the hypertrophic cell layer of the physis. Type III fractures account for approximately 10% of physeal injuries. A Salter–Harris type IV fracture line originates at the articular surface, crosses the epiphysis, extends through the full thickness of the physis, and exits through a segment of the metaphysis.

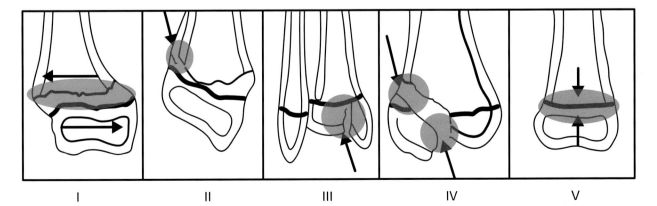

Figure 29.1 Salter–Harris classification system with fractures I–V. Note that increasing Salter–Harris classification system number carries a greater risk of growth arrest due to physeal injury.

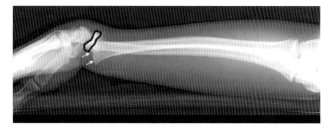

Figure 29.2 Lateral forearm and wrist with a Salter–Harris type I fracture of the distal radius. Note that the epiphysis (outlined in black) of the distal radius has been displaced into a dorsal position relative to the physis (arrows) and metaphysis of the bone. The clinician can confuse the epiphyseal in this radiograph with a carpal bone, entirely missing the growth plate fracture.

Type IV injuries are seen most commonly at the lower end of the humerus. Type IV injuries represent approximately 10% of all physeal fractures. Salter–Harris type V injuries are the least frequent of physeal fractures, accounting for less than 1% of growth plate injuries; this type of fracture is by the far the most likely injury to result in focal bone growth arrest. These injuries occur most frequently at the knee or ankle, and are the result of a severe abduction or adduction injury that transmits profound compressive forces across the physis. This resultant axial compression crushes the physis, and

specifically injures the cells of the reserve and proliferative zones (Figure 29.2).

A Salter–Harris type I injury is most appropriately managed with splint immobilization, intermittent icing, elevation, and referral to an orthopedic surgeon for re-evaluation. Type II injuries, if there is no angulation or significant displacement of the fracture fragment, can be similarly managed. Type III and IV fractures usually require orthopedic consultation with near-perfect re-alignment of the epiphyseal fracture fragment for both blood supply maintenance and joint congruity. Type V injuries similarly require orthopedic consultation with casting followed by limited use of the involved extremity. In certain instances, any type Salter–Harris fracture may require reduction and/or realignment of the fracture fragment; infact, the patient noted in this case required reduction of the epiphysis prior to discharge.

Further reading

1 Della-Giustina K, Della-Giustina DA. Emergency department evaluation and treatment of pediatric orthopedic injuries. *Emerg Med Clin North Am* 1999;**17**: 895–922.
2 England SP, Sundberg S. Management of common pediatric fractures. *Pediatr Clin North Am* 1996;**43**:991–1012.
3 Kaeding CC, Whitehead R. Musculoskeletal injuries in adolescents. *Primary Care Clin Office Pract* 1998;**25**: 211–23.

Case 30 | **Raccoon eyes**

Answer: D
Diagnosis: Periorbital hematoma
Discussion: "Raccoon eyes," depicted in the picture on page 20, are also known as periorbital hematoma and is often a sign of basilar skull fracture. These injuries are associated with a high morbidity and mortality, and should be diagnosed in a timely fashion. Basilar skull fractures are linear fractures at the base of the skull and often occur through the temporal bone leading to bleeding into the middle ear and hemotympanum. These fractures are also often associated with a torn dura, and patients are at risk for developing meningitis. Patients with basilar fractures may complain of vertigo, tinnitus, dizziness, and decreased hearing. In addition to periorbital hematoma, other signs of basilar skull fracture include mastoid ecchymoses (Battle's sign or retroauricular hematoma), hemotympanum, cerebral spinal fluid rhinorrhea or otorrhea, and seventh nerve palsy. Periorbital and mastoid ecchymoses may take a few hours to appear and may be absent during the initial evaluation.

A study examining the positive predictive values of the above clinical signs found unilateral periorbital hematoma to have a positive predictive value for skull base fractures of 90%, bilateral periorbital hematoma of 70%, and Battle's

sign of 100%. The positive predictive values for acute intracranial lesions (including subdural hematoma, brain contusion, pneumocephalus, epidural hematoma, and brain swelling) were 85% for unilateral periorbital hematoma, 68% for bilateral periorbital hematoma, and 66% for Battle's sign. This suggests the clinical signs of raccoon eyes and Battle sign have very high positive predictive values for both skull fractures and intracranial injury.

Those patients who are suspected of having a skull fracture should undergo emergent computed tomography (CT) scan of the head to evaluate for intracranial injury and to define the fracture. Skull radiographs do not detect basilar skull fractures well. Patients with a basilar fracture should be admitted for observation. Antibiotics may be considered for the prevention of meningitis.

Further reading

1 Pretto Flores L, De Almeida CS, Casulari LA. Positive predictive values of selected clinical signs associated with skull base fractures. *J Neurosurg Sci* 2000;**44**(2):77–82.
2 Herbella FA, Mudo M, Delmonti C, *et al.* "Raccoon eyes" (periorbital haematoma) as a sign of skull base fracture. *Injury* 2001; **32**(10):745–7.

Case 31 | **Chest pain and a confounding electrocardiogram pattern**

Answer: B

Diagnosis: Left bundle branch block and acute myocardial infarction

Discussion: The electrocardiograph (ECG) in this case demonstrates a normal sinus rhythm and a left bundle branch block (LBBB) with excessive discordant ST segment elevation in leads V2, V3, and V4, as well as concordant ST segment elevation in leads V5 and V6 – the findings are consistent with anterolateral ST-elevation myocardial infarction (STEMI) in an LBBB pattern.

Patients with LBBB and acute myocardial infarction (AMI) are at an increased risk of experiencing a poor outcome; these patients should be rapidly and aggressively managed. In patients with AMI, both the pre-existing and the new-onset LBBB are clinical markers for a significantly worsened prognosis in terms of higher mortality, lower left ventricular ejection fraction, and increased incidence of cardiovascular

complications. The new development of LBBB in the setting of AMI suggests proximal occlusion of the left anterior descending artery. A prior history of LBBB in patients with AMI places the patient at risk of cardiogenic shock due to the often associated depressed left ventricular function. Despite this increased risk of poor outcome, patients with LBBB less often receive fibrinolytic therapy. These same patients show significant benefit when treated with thrombolytic therapy; the presence of a new LBBB in the setting of AMI is considered an indication for pharmacologic thrombolysis.

LBBB is a confounding pattern which reduces the ECG's ability to detect acute coronary syndrome (ACS). A new, or *presumably new*, LBBB is strongly suggestive of ACS when noted in the appropriate clinical presentation. Pre-existing LBBB, however, shares many ECG similarities to various ECG findings of ACS. In the normal LBBB presentation, the right-sided precordial leads demonstrate ST segment elevation and

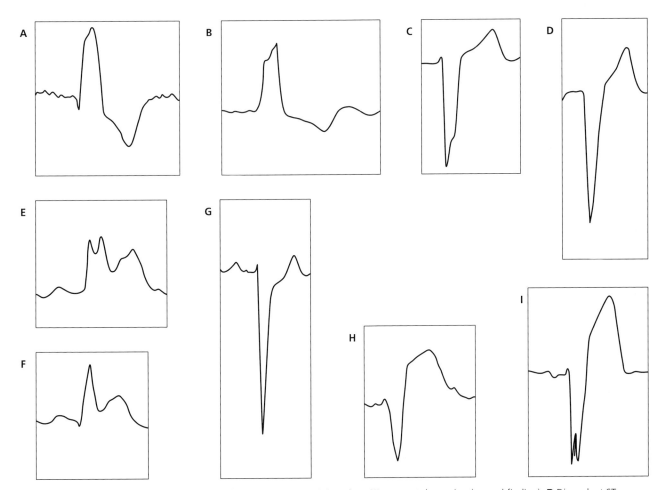

Figure 31.1 Rule of appropriate discordance in the LBBB pattern. **A** Discordant ST segment depression (normal finding). **B** Discordant ST segment depression (normal finding). **C and D** Discordant ST segment elevation less than 5 mm (normal finding). **E and F** Concordant ST segment elevation (abnormal finding, consistent with AMI). **G** Concordant ST segment depression (abnormal finding, consistent with AMI). **H and I** Excessive, discordant ST segment elevation greater than 5 mm (abnormal finding, consistent with ACS).

tall, upright T waves; these T waves mimic prominent T waves seen in STEMI. The QS pattern of LBBB in these leads resembles the Q waves seen in infarction. Depressed ST segments with T wave inversions are seen in some or all of the lateral leads (V5, V6, I, and aVL) in LBBB; both of these resemble ischemic changes seen in ACS. Yet these findings in LBBB are merely expressions of the "rule of appropriate discordance."

The "rule of appropriate discordance" describes the appropriate ST segment deflections relative to the major portion of the QRS complex. The ST segment and T wave vectors are expectedly discordant, or opposite in direction, to the major vector of the QRS complex in those leads. Sgarbossa and colleagues reported three ECG predictors of AMI in the presence of LBBB, including: (1) ST segment elevation of at least 1 mm that is concordant with the QRS complex; (2) ST segment depression of at least 1 mm in leads V1, V2, or V3; and (3) ST

segment elevation of at least 5 mm that is discordant with the QRS complex. Ultimately, the approach to the patient with LBBB and possible myocardial infarction remains complicated; diagnostic adjuncts to the history and physical examination (e.g., serial ECGs, comparison with prior ECGs, echocardiography, serum cardiac marker measurement, etc.) should be liberally employed when the ECG does not show obvious evidence of AMI as noted by the Sgarbossa criteria.

Further reading

1 Sgarbossa EB, Pinski SL, Barbagelata A, *et al.* Electrocardiographic diagnosis of evolving acute myocardial infarction in the presence of left bundle branch block. *New Engl J Med* 1996; **334**:481–7.
2 Rosner MH, Brady WJ. The ECG diagnosis of acute myocardial infarction in the presence of left bundle branch block. *Am J Emerg Med* 1998;**16**(7):697–700.

Case 32 | **Eye pain in a contact lens wearer**

Answer: C
Diagnosis: Corneal ulcer secondary to *Pseudomonas*
Discussion: The photograph on page 21 shows a large corneal ulcer depicted by a fluffy stromal infiltrate and an overlying epithelial defect. There are several etiologies of ulcerative keratitis, but infectious causes should be presumed until proven otherwise. Bacterial corneal ulceration is the most common infectious etiology and often sight-threatening. Virulent pathogens can have a rapid onset and progression that, left untreated, may progress to perforation. Less frequently, infectious causes may be fungal, viral, and protozoan.

Case history is important in determining the cause of corneal ulceration. The most frequent risk factor for corneal ulcer in the United States is contact lens wear. This risk increases significantly in patients who sleep in their lenses overnight. Traumatic ocular injuries, particularly from

vegetable matter, increase the suspicion of a fungal etiology. Corneal scrapings for Gram stain and culture are paramount in the management of corneal ulcers.

Initial therapy with a broad-spectrum antibiotic is recommended until the offending organism is identified in culture. Severe cases may require fortified antibiotics. Contact lens wearers must discontinue their lens wear. Ophthalmologic consultation is required for corneal ulcers since these patients require close outpatient follow-up.

Further reading

1 Schein OD, Glynn RJ, Poggio EC, *et al.* The relative risk of ulcerative keratitis among users of daily-wear and extended-wear soft contact lenses. A case–control study. Microbial Keratitis Study Group. *New Engl J Med* 1989;**321**(12):773–8.
2 Ma JJ, Dohlman CH. Mechanisms of corneal ulceration. *Ophthalmol Clin North Am* 2002;**15**(1):27–33.

Case 33 | **Heel pain following a fall**

Answer: B
Diagnosis: Displaced calcaneus fracture
Discussion: Calcaneus fractures are the most common tarsal bone fractures. To induce a calcaneus fracture, a significant amount of force must be transmitted. Calcaneus fractures are usually a result of an axial load, commonly occurring after a fall from a significant height when landing in a standing

position. They are part of the spectrum of axial loading injuries to the lower extremity, which can include calcaneus fractures, pylon (plafond) fractures, tibial plateau fractures, femur fractures, and fracture–dislocation of the hip. Greater than 20% of calcaneus fractures have accompanying lumbar spine compression fractures, so all patients with calcaneus fractures should have screening lumbar spine radiographs.

Foot X-rays to evaluate for calcaneus fractures can be difficult to interpret. Subtle, non-displaced calcaneus fractures are often missed on a routine foot series. Close examination of the lateral view for changes in the cortical and trabecular bone often reveals subtle fractures. Increased density of markings in the trabecular architecture may be the only sign of a compression fracture. Dedicated axial views of the calcaneus, obtained with the X-ray beam projected perpendicular to the long axis of the calcaneus, can improve sensitivity. Boehler's angle determined by the angle formed by two straight lines: one drawn along the superior surface of the posterior tuberosity of the calcaneus to the superior tip of the subtalar articular surface and the other connecting the superior tip of the subtalar articular surface with the apex of the anterior surface of the calcaneus is normally between 20 and 40 degrees. The majority of calcaneus fractures have a decrease in Boehler's angle to less than 20 degrees as shown in Figure 33.1. Computerized tomography (CT) scanning helps in pre-operative management of complex calcaneus fractures to differentiate extra-articular from intra-articular fractures and should also be considered in the patient with ongoing pain, inability to ambulate, and normal plain radiographs.

Calcaneus fractures are classified similarly to as all other fractures, and the type of fracture dictates subsequent management. A careful search for evidence of open fracture must be done. Non-displaced fractures can be treated with immobilization and orthopedic follow-up. Fractures displaced more than 3 mm, comminuted fractures, and intra-articular fractures (extending into the subtalar joint) need operative management for open reduction and internal fixation of the fracture fragments. The post-injury course can be complicated by compartment syndrome (suggested by extreme swelling at the plantar arch), nonunion, chronic pain, and arthritis of the subtalar joint.

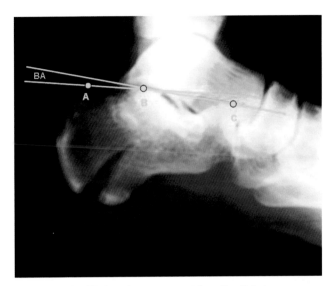

Figure 33.1 Boehler's angle measurement from the clinical case. Two lines are drawn, one from the posterior calcaneal tubercle (A) to the most superior point of the calcaneus (B), the other from the anterior calcaneal tubercle (C) to the most superior part of the calcaneus (B). Boehler's angle (BA) represents the acute angle of intersection between these two lines and is normally between 20 and 40 degrees. An angle of less than 20 degrees, such as in this case, suggests a calcaneal fracture.

Further reading

1 Germann CA, Perron AD, Miller MD, *et al.* Orthopedic pitfalls in the ED: calcaneal fractures. *Am J Emerg Med* 2004;**22**(7):607–11.
2 Chen MY, Bohrer SP, Kelley TF. Boehler's angle: a reappraisal. *Ann Emerg Med* 1991;**20**(2):122–4.

Case 34 | **FAST evaluation following trauma**

Answer: E
Diagnosis: Intraperitoneal free fluid (i.e. blood)
Discussion: The focused assessment by sonography in trauma (FAST) evaluates for free fluid in the potential spaces of the trunk. Varying views and degrees of complexity have been advocated in performing this examination. These can be simplified and unified if it is remembered that the exam is trying to detect abnormal collections of fluid as they will be found in a supine patient. The potential spaces that are evaluated in the right upper (RUQ) and left upper quadrants (LUQ) are the pleural, subphrenic and perirenal. The perirenal space is usually referred to as the hepatorenal or Morison's pouch in the RUQ, and the splenorenal in the LUQ. The colic gutters, sometimes included in the FAST, are

anatomical extensions of the perirenal spaces; therefore, a complete exam of the inferior extent of the perirenal spaces will effectively include these spaces. The pericardial space is evaluated from a subxiphoid (also known as "subcostal") window, or, if necessary (i.e. due to abdominal wall trauma, abdominal pain, or protuberance) via parasternal views. The final potential spaces to be evaluated are in the pelvis: the retrovesicular space in the male and the rectouterine space in the female ("pouch of Douglas"). These are the most dependent spaces in the entire abdominal cavity. However, in most cases of blunt trauma, the sources of peritoneal blood are the solid organs and vascular structures of the upper abdomen, which will fill the dependent spaces of the upper abdomen before reaching the level of the pelvic brim

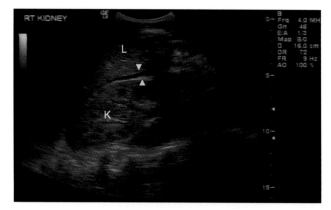

Figure 34.1 Right upper quadrant view (K: kidney; L: liver).

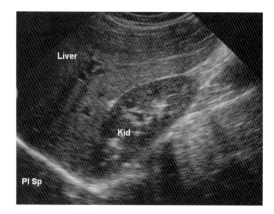

Figure 34.2 Normal right upper quadrant view (Kid: kidney; Pl Sp: pleural space).

and draining into the pelvis. For this reason, blood is much more frequently found in upper abdominal locations than in the pelvis in the supine patient.

Figure 34.1 shows the RUQ view from the case. Figure 34.2 shows a normal RUQ demonstrating all three of the spaces discussed above. The diaphragm (long arrows) divides the pleural space from the subphrenic space. Morison's pouch (short arrows) is seen between the liver and kidney. In the absence of abnormal collections of free fluid, Morison's pouch and the diaphragm are strongly echogenic, therefore appearing white on the image. In Figure 34.1, the dark anechoic stripe (arrowheads) is caused by fluid in this potential space. In more than 50% of cases of positive FAST exams, free fluid is seen in Morison's pouch. Some authorities have made the *a priori* estimate that a small stripe in Morison's pouch represents about 250 mL of intraperitoneal fluid. However, accurate operative assessment of intraperitoneal free fluid volumes is not possible. Studies using diagnostic peritoneal lavage as a model suggest that the volume needed to be reliably detected in Morison's pouch is closer to 650 mL of free fluid. Placing the patient in Trendelenburg reduces this volume by 33% to about 450 mL.

In the case of this trauma patient, the sonographic evidence of hemoperitoneum with hemodynamic instability mandates immediate transfer to the operating room for exploratory laparotomy. Although computed tomography

(CT) scanning is superior to sonography in identifying solid organ injury, it has several disadvantages. These include the removal of the patient from the resuscitation area, the use of intravenous and oral contrast agents, commitment of significant manpower resources, and expense. In this case it would also delay the definitive care of a patient already in hemorrhagic shock. The transfusion of blood products is a critical action, but allowing the patient to remain in the emergency department for serial exams is not a viable option because of the strong evidence for a life-threatening injury. Finally, diagnostic peritoneal lavage in this case is not warranted since the FAST exam has already demonstrated the presence of intraperitoneal fluid.

Further reading

1 Rose J. Ultrasound in abdominal trauma. *Emerg Med Clin North Am* 2004;**22**:581–99.

2 Jehle D, Guarino J, Karamanoukian H. Emergency department ultrasound in the evaluation of blunt abdominal trauma. *Am J Em Med* 1993;**11**(4):342–6.

3 Rozycki GS, Ochsner MG, Feliciano DV, Thomas B, *et al.* Early detection of hemoperitoneum by ultrasound examination of the right upper quadrant: a multicenter study. *J Trauma* 1998; **45**(5):878–83.

4 Abrams BJ, Sukumvanich P, Seibel R, Moscati R, *et al.* Ultrasound for the detection of intraperitoneal fluid: the role of trendelenburg positioning. *Am J Emerg Med* 1999;**17**(2):117–20.

Case 35 | **Skin lesion in a heroin addict**

Answer: B
Diagnosis: Skin popping
Discussion: This case demonstrates skin findings consistent with cellulitis and multiple ulcerations suggestive of skin popping. Upon further questioning, the patient admitted to

heroin use through subcutaneous injections. Figure 35.1 shows the fifth proximal phalanx projecting through the skin at a site of one of her skin popping ulcerations. The patient recalled that she had fallen on her hand approximately 1 month prior.

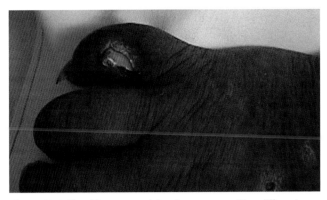

Figure 35.1 The skin popper of the chapter case with a different view of her hand revealing the proximal phalanx of her fifth digit protruding through the abscess.

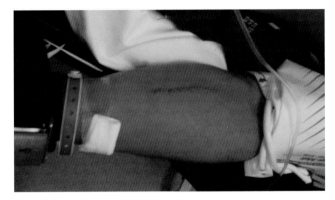

Figure 35.2 Characteristic "track" marks of an intravenous drug abuser.

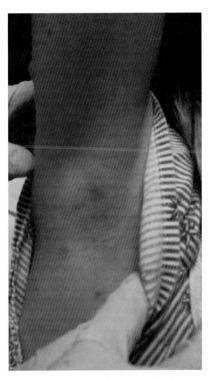

Figure 35.3 Injection marks within the axilla of an intravenous drug abuser. The axilla was utilized to avoid detection.

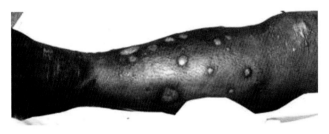

Figure 35.4 Characteristic multiple abscesses on the leg of a skin popper.

Skin popping is performed by drug abusers usually after intravenous access is no longer available secondary to scelerosis, thrombosis, dissection, or overlying infection of their veins shown in Figure 35.2. The techniques employed are often not sterile and involve the deposition of not only the abused drug but also contaminates, such as particulate matter and bacteria, subcutaneously. Skin popping often results in abscess formation and cellulitis. Skin popping is a risk factor for developing deadly clostridial infections including tetanus, botulism, and necrotizing fasciitis. *Staphylococcus*, *Streptococcus*, and *Bacillus* species have also been isolated from these wounds.

Parenteral drug abusers are known to use many different routes of injection to obtain their fix. Careful physical examination should be performed on all suspected drug abusers. Grand central station is a rare practice that involves the injection of illicit drugs directly into the heart using the sub-xiphoid approach. Pocketing involves the injection of drugs into the subclavian vein using a supraclavicular approach through the pocket palpated between the clavicle and the neck.

Further reading

1 Binswanger IA, Kral AH, Bluthenthal RN, *et al*. High prevalence of abscesses and cellulitis among community-recruited injection drug users in San Francisco. *Clin Infect Dis* 2000;**30**(3):579–81.
2 Brown PD, Ebright JR. Skin and soft tissue infections in injection drug users. *Curr Infect Dis Rep* 2002;**4**(5): 415–19.

Case 36 | **Young athlete with back pain**

Answer: D

Diagnosis: Pars defect at L5

Discussion: Lower back pain in a young athletic patient is a common phenomenon. Often, these complaints are non-specific. Substantial decrease in performance and recurrence of symptoms can be important historical elements.

Pars defect (spondylolysis) is a defect of the posterior bony spine consisting of an interruption in the vertebral arch between the superior and inferior articular processes (*pars interarticularis*). The majority (90%) of cases occur at L5 although other lumbar vertebrae may be involved. It is most commonly bilateral but unilateral defects are observed. The pathophysiology of spondylolysis appears to center around repeated trauma to the pars interarticularis giving rise to stress fractures of the arch. Preexisting spinal abnormalities such as spina bifida occulta are associated with a higher risk of spondylolysis. Some believe that there is a genetic component to spondylolysis but this remains controversial.

Spondylolysis is more common in men and young athletes who participate in sports such as football, soccer, gymnastics, wrestling, and tennis. The disorder is often asymptomatic but can be associated with significant morbidity. Patients with bilateral spondylolysis can progress to spondylolisthesis – a forward slippage of the adjacent vertebrae.

Evaluation in the emergency department should include a thorough neurological exam to assess for any significant deficits, which might signify a more serious lesion. Careful attention should be paid to range of motion abnormalities. Often pain on extension or rotation of the lumbar spine may be the only finding on exam. Plain radiographs of the lumbar spine, consisting of anteroposterior (AP), lateral, and oblique views should be obtained. On a normal oblique view, the posterior spinal elements form a "Scotty dog" appearance (see Figure 36.1). A fracture line through the neck of the Scotty dog signifies a disruption of the pars interarticularis. Magnetic resonance imaging (MRI), computerized axial tomography (CT) scanning and single photon emission computed tomography (SPECT) can be useful adjuncts for diagnosis. Management in the emergency department includes analgesia and activity limitation. Consultation with a spine specialist may be necessary if symptoms persist despite activity limitation. Bracing and surgery may be needed if there is no response to conservative management.

Further reading

1 Bono CM. Low-back pain in athletes. *J Bone Joint Surg Am* 2004;**86**-A(2):382–96.
2 Greenan TJ. Diagnostic imaging of sports-related spinal disorders. *Clin Sports Med* 1993;**12**(3):487–505.

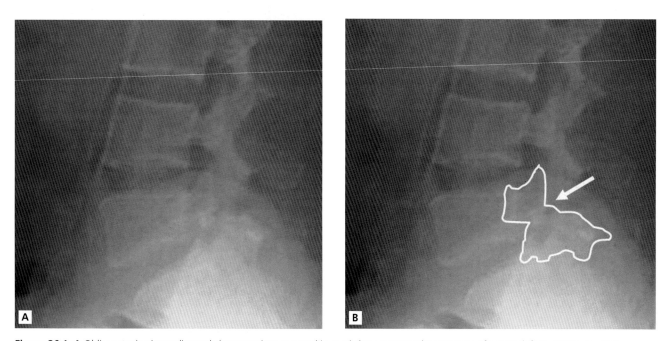

Figure 36.1 A Oblique projection radiograph (same patient as noted in case) demonstrates the presence of a pars defect. **B** This resembles a Scotty dog with a collar (drawn with arrow).

Case 37 | **Skin lesions in a comatose patient**

Answer: C

Diagnosis: Rhabdomyolysis

Discussion: Rhabdomyolysis is defined as the breakdown of skeletal muscle due to injury. Muscle injury can occur from multiple causes. This muscle damage may result in potential life-threatening complications including myoglobinuric acute renal failure, hyperkalemia, disseminated intravascular coagulation, and compartment syndrome.

The primary laboratory test that indicates the presence of rhabdomyolysis is an elevated serum creatine phosphokinase (CPK). The CPK-MM isoenzyme predominates in rhabdomyolysis, comprising at least 98% of the total value. The other laboratory indicator frequently seen in rhabdomyolysis is myoglobinuria. Myoglobin functions as an oxygen store in skeletal muscle fibers. As myoglobin is released into the circulation from damaged muscle cells it produces visible pigmenturia (classically a "coca-cola" colored urine) that can be misidentified as hematuria. If patient has what appears to be marked hematuria, but the microscopic examination of the urine fails to demonstrate any red blood cells, then myoglobinuria should be suspected. Other important laboratory findings in rhabdomyolysis include hyperkalemia, hypocalcemia, hyperphosphatemia, hyperuricemia, and elevated levels of other muscle enzymes including lactate dehydrogenase and aminotransferases.

There is an extensive list of causes of rhabdomyolysis. Rare hereditary causes of rhabdomyolysis consist primarily of various enzyme defects. There are numerous acquired causes, and include traumatic, ischemic, metabolic, infectious, inflammatory, and toxic causes. Although the causes of rhabdomyolysis are diverse, the pathogenesis follows a final common pathway, ultimately leading to muscle necrosis and release of muscle components into the circulation. The common pathogenesis of all disease processes causing rhabdomyolysis is an acute rise in the cytosolic and mitochondrial calcium concentration in affected muscle cells, which sets off a chain of events that ultimately results in muscle cell necrosis.

The clinical features of rhabdomyolysis are quite variable depending on the cause of the rhabdomyolysis. Muscle pain and weakness may be the presenting complaints in those patients who are alert. Muscle tenderness may be noted on examination. Patients who are comatose may have only subtle findings on examination. The case presented demonstrated a patient whose only physical finding was skin breakdown over pressure points noted in the pictures on page 24 (the patient was found lying on his side). Figure 37.1, for example, demonstrates a comatose phenobarbital overdose patient who had subtle skin changes in the area of her buttocks associated with pressure necrosis and underlying rhabdomyolysis.

The complications of rhabdomyolysis are due to the local effects of muscle injury and the systemic effects of released

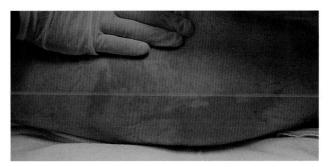

Figure 37.1 Subtle skin changes in the buttocks region of a comatose phenobarbital overdose associated with pressure necrosis. The patient was subsequently found to have marked underlying rhabdomyolysis. This case demonstrates the importance of exposing and completely examining the skin of all comatose patients presenting to the emergency department.

muscle components. Hyperkalemia can precipitate dysrhythmias and cardiac arrest. Hyperkalemia may be potentiated by associated hypocalcemia. Hyperkalemia should be recognized early and treated with appropriate pharmacologic therapies (i.e. intravenous fluids, albuterol, sodium bicarbonate, insulin with glucose, calcium, and ion exchange resins) and potentially emergent dialysis. Compartment syndrome can develop in acute rhabdomyolysis as muscle swelling occurs within a tight fascial compartment, leading to compression of vessels and nerves. Prolonged ischemia and infarction of muscle tissue can result in replacement of muscle by inelastic fibrous tissue and severe contractures (i.e. Volkmann's contracture). The treatment of suspected compartment syndrome is urgent decompression by open fasciotomy. Acute renal failure is the most common complication of rhabdomyolysis, occurring in approximately 30% of patients. Prevention of acute renal failure involves maintenance of circulating blood volume by adequate fluid replacement to assure a urine output of approximately 1.0 mL/kg/hour. Mannitol may be considered to maintain a diuresis. Alkalinization of the urine by administering an intravenous infusion of sodium bicarbonate has been suggested since acidic urine favors myoglobin nephrotoxicity. However, this therapy is controversial since no strong evidence exists that this therapy alters the clinical outcome and it may in fact induce further hypocalcemia.

Further reading

1 Coco TJ, Klasner AE. Drug-induced rhabdomyolysis. *Curr Opin Pediatr* 2004;**16**(2):206–10.
2 Malinoski DJ, Slater MS, Mullins RJ. Crush injury and rhabdomyolysis. *Crit Care Clin* 2004;**20**(1):171–92.

Case 38 | Chest pain with sudden cardiac death

Answer: D

Diagnosis: Polymorphic ventricular tachycardia and QT prolongation

Discussion: The rhythm strip demonstrates polymorphic ventricular tachycardia (PVT) with a polymorphous QRS complex; note the variation in the morphology and amplitude of the QRS complex – it appears to twist around a fixed point. This rhythm is an example of a specific type of PVT, torsade de pointes (TdP). The ECG demonstrates normal sinus rhythm with prolonged QT-interval and T-wave inversions in leads II, III, aVf, V2, V3, V4, V5, and V6 – consistent with an acute coronary syndrome.

Long QT syndrome (LQTS) is an electrophysiologic cardiac disorder in which the repolarization phase of the ventricular action potential is lengthened. It is manifested as a prolongation of the QT interval on the surface ECG and is clinically significant in that it can precipitate the development of PVT and sudden cardiac death. Congenital and acquired forms of LQTS are encountered, the former due to abnormalities in transmembrane ion channels and the latter due to multiple causes including medications and toxins, electrolyte imbalance, bradycardia, central nervous system event, acute coronary syndrome, autonomic neuropathy, and the human immunodeficiency virus.

Patients with LQTS may present with a variety of symptoms, ranging from mild dizziness to syncope or, in the extreme, sudden cardiac death – likely resulting from TdP, a form of PVT that occurs in the setting of QT-interval prolongation. TdP is recognized on a surface ECG as progressive, complete 180 degree twisting of the QRS complexes around an imaginary baseline. Because TdP is usually limited to 10–12 beats and terminates spontaneously, patients may complain of only mild dizziness or may even be asymptomatic. Syncope and sudden cardiac death can result from rapidly recurring or sustained episodes of TdP which ultimately degenerate into ventricular fibrillation. Clinical presentation: patients with LQTS may present to the emergency department (ED) with a variety of symptoms, ranging from mild dizziness to syncope or, in the extreme, sudden cardiac death. These symptoms are all due to TdP, a form of PVT that occurs in the setting of QT-interval prolongation. It is recognized on a surface ECG as progressive, complete 180 degree twisting of the QRS complexes around an imaginary baseline. Because torsades is usually limited to 10–12 beats and terminates spontaneously, patients may complain of only mild dizziness or may even be asymptomatic. Syncope and sudden cardiac death can result from rapidly recurring or sustained episodes of torsades which ultimately degenerate into ventricular fibrillation.

The diagnosis of LQTS is made via the combination of symptoms, family history, and ECG abnormality, T-wave

Table 38.1 Determination of the corrected QT interval

Calculated determination
Bazett formula – calculates the QT interval corrected for heart rate by dividing the QT interval by the square root of the R–R interval
$QTc = QT/[R-R]^{0.5}$

Rapid bedside determination
For rates between 60 and 100 bpm, the QT interval may be rapidly and reliably corrected for the particular rate. If the QT interval is less than one-half the accompanying R–R interval, the QT interval is appropriate for that rate.

alternans, and U-waves. A QT interval which is prolonged, usually greater than 450 m/second, is considered abnormal and potentially suggestive of the syndrome. For example, a QTc interval greater than 440 m/second places a patient at a 2–3 higher risk for sudden death than does a QTc interval of less than 440 m/second. The QTc interval may be calculated using the Bazett formula (Table 38.1) or via comparative measurements to the accompanying R–R interval – a QT interval which is less than one-half the accompanying R–R interval is considered normal.

The management of the patient with LQTS involves immediate therapy of active dysrhythmia followed by recognition of the syndrome; further management of LQTS then involves a correction of any precipitating issues, such as electrolyte abnormality, bradycardia, medication adverse effect, acute coronary ischemia, etc. Emergent treatment involves electrical cardioversion or defibrillation for the patient presenting in sustained TdP. Treatment is then needed to prevent the recurrence of TdP, which may involve correcting any electrolyte abnormality, removing any offending agent possibly prolonging the QT interval, and instituting temporary transvenous overdrive cardiac pacing if necessary. The acquired forms of LQTS generally do not require any long-term treatment as correction of the offending issue is usually adequate. In patients with acquired LQTS secondary to bradycardia, implantation of a permanent pacemaker is usually effective. Long-term treatment of congenital LQTS, however, is essential to prevent recurrences of TdP, including beta-adrenergic blocking agents and implantable pacemaker-cardioverter-defibrillator.

Further reading

1 Schwartz PJ. Idiopathic long QT syndrome: progress and questions. *Am Heart J* 1985;**2**:399–411.
2 Schwartz PJ, Moss AJ, Vincent GM, *et al.* Diagnostic criteria for the long QT syndrome: an update. *Circulation* 1993; **88**:782–4.

Case 39 | **Fall on an outstretched hand with wrist pain**

Answer: C

Diagnosis: Scaphoid fracture

Discussion: One of the most common, and yet dangerous, diagnoses made in the injured extremity is the *wrist sprain*. Wrist sprains certainly do occur but the diagnosis should only be entertained after careful physical and radiographic examinations have ruled out fracture and dislocation in this region. In fact, the diagnosis *wrist sprain* is one of exclusion. Proper diagnosis of the wrist injury is dependent on a thorough knowledge of the topographical anatomy of the wrist and careful, systematic evaluation of the extremity and appropriate radiographs. Fractures of the scaphoid account for 60–70% of all diagnosed carpal injuries. Unfortunately, fracture of the scaphoid bone is a frequently missed diagnosis. Radiographic findings are either subtle or absent making the diagnosis difficult in the absence of a thorough, well-performed clinical examination. Accurate early diagnosis is critical as the morbidity associated with a missed or late diagnosis is significant, including chronic pain, reduced functional ability, and osteonecrosis.

The classic history for scaphoid fracture is the fall on the outstretched hand – the so-called FOOSH mechanism. The patient generally has immediate pain yet has little or no soft tissue swelling; it is not uncommon for the patient to continue his or her activity, only seeking medical care at a later time.

In that the demonstration of specific point tenderness within the carpus is the most important diagnostic test in assessing injuries to the wrist, it is critical that clinicians be comfortable with the anatomy of this area. The anatomic snuffbox is the area between the tendons of the first and third dorsal compartments on the radial side of the wrist. This area is best palpated by bringing the thumb into radial abduction, defining the hollow situated between the extensor pollicus longus, the abductor pollicus longus, and extensor pollicus brevis. The radial styloid is palpable at the base of the snuffbox and the body of the scaphoid is palpable in the depths of this area. On the palmar aspect, the distal wrist crease is the visible landmark which defines the underlying anatomy. At the intersection of the flexor carpi radialis tendon and the radial wrist crease, the scaphoid tuberosity is palpable as a bony prominence at the base of the thenar muscles. Proper palpation during physical examination, however, will exacerbate pain, prompting the physician to obtain the proper films. The patient's degree of swelling, discomfort, and motion loss will be variable. Palpation of the scaphoid bone in the anatomic snuffbox is most reliable diagnostic maneuver; direct palpation of the scaphoid tuberosity from the palmar aspect should also demonstrate tenderness. An additional maneuver involves an axial load placed upon the first digit in extension; with scaphoid fracture, such a load transfers force onto the injured bone, producing pain.

Although the diagnosis of scaphoid fracture is suggested by the history and physical examination, it is confirmed only by

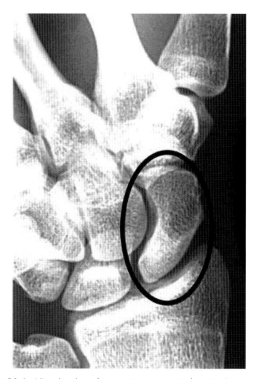

Figure 39.1 AP wrist view demonstrates a normal appearing scaphoid bone (black oval circle) with normal relationships to adjacent carpal structures.

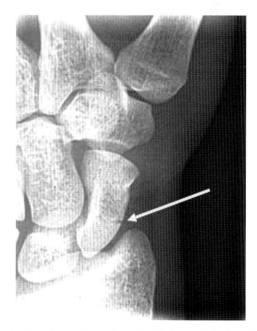

Figure 39.2 Navicular view of the patient in Figure 39.1 demonstrates a fracture in the mid portion (arrow), or waist, of the scaphoid. Note that this fracture was not apparent on the standard AP wrist view.

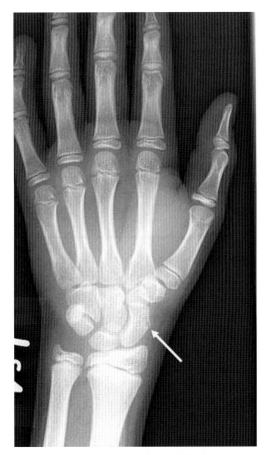

radiographic evaluation – in a majority of cases. As with most orthopedic radiographic evaluations, a minimum of two views oriented perpendicular to one another are appropriate (the anteroposterior and lateral views); additionally, an oblique view provides yet another important perspective. Supplemental views, such as the navicular view (a focused image of the scaphoid oriented in an anteroposterior (AP) fashion with the long axis of the bone parallel to the film), provides additional radiographic assistance. Even with appropriate films and interpretation, these fractures can be subtle and difficult to see. A significant percentage of these fractures will not be visible on any view at initial presentation.

Most suspected scaphoid injuries should be treated initially as though a fracture exists, that is splint and refer to a clinician for repeat evaluation. Since a number of these fractures are not radiographically detectable on initial presentation, most patients with an appropriate injury mechanism and examination (i.e. snuffbox tenderness) should be treated with a thumb spica splint and evaluated by a clinician in 10–14 days. Strict adherence to this policy will ensure that any fracture with subtle or absent radiographic initial findings will still be appropriately treated without delay. Undiagnosed, and therefore improperly treated, scaphoid fracture is complicated by chronic pain, reduced functional ability, and early arthritis due to the ischemic necrosis and malunion.

Figure 39.3 Scaphoid fracture (arrow) in a child. The patient presented with wrist pain after a FOOSH mechanism. Examination demonstrated tenderness with no soft tissue swelling in the anatomic snuffbox; importantly, no tenderness was noted at the growth plate of the distal radius which is the more likely fracture location in this particular patient population.

Further reading

1 Brooks S, Wluka AE, Stuckey S, Cicuttini F. The management of scaphoid fractures. *J Sci Med Sport* 2005;**8**:181–9.
2 Foes B, Speake, P, Body R. Best evidence topic report. Magnetic resonance imaging or bone scintigraphy in the diagnosis of plain X ray occult scaphoid fractures. *Emerg Med J* 2005;**22**:434–5.
3 Barnaby W. Fractures and dislocations of the wrist. *Emerg Med Clin North Am* 1992;**10**:133–49.

Case 40 | **Necrotic skin lesion**

Answer: C
Diagnosis: Pyoderma gangrenosum
Discussion: Pyoderma gangrenosum (PG) is an uncommon inflammatory skin disease of unknown etiology. It typically presents on the trunk or lower extremities of adults 40–60 years old. Women may be slightly more often affected than men. Approximately 50% of cases of PG are associated with one of the following four main categories of systemic disease:

(1) inflammatory bowel disease (i.e. Crohn's disease and ulcerative colitis)
(2) hematological disorders (i.e. acute lymphoid and myeloid leukemias, myeloma)

(3) rheumatological conditions (i.e. rheumatoid arthritis and lupus erythematosus)
(4) hepatic disease (i.e. chronic active hepatitis, primary biliary cirrhosis).

PG usually presents initially as a small pustule or nodule that patients often attribute to a spider bite. The lesion then typically enlarges and ulcerates. The resulting ulcer classically has a distinct violaceous "rolled-up" margin that is elevated, undermined, and may be covered with necrotic debris and small abscesses. There may be an associated purulent and hemorrhagic exudate. The ulcer may be a few centimeters wide or may span the length of an entire limb. PG lesions typically heal with a characteristic slightly depressed, "punched out" scar.

Patients with PG may also complain of fever, malaise, gastrointestinal symptoms, and arthralgias. The work-up of a patient with an ulcer should be guided by the physical findings as well as comorbidities. Before a diagnosis of PG can be made, other causes of ulcers must be ruled out. Tissue biopsy and tissue culture, rather than simply a swab culture of the ulcer base, are the most definitive ways to rule out other causes of ulcers, which include (but are not limited to) vascular, traumatic, infectious (i.e. bacterial, fungal, and atypical mycobacterial), inflammatory (i.e. vasculitic), and neoplastic (i.e. basal or squamous cell carcinoma). Performing a wedge-shaped incisional biopsy from peri-lesional skin toward the center of the ulcer, traversing the ulcer edge, is recommended; if this is not possible, several punch biopsies of various areas of the ulcers can be performed.

PG is treated with immunosuppressive agents, most commonly intralesional or oral steroids. Debridement is contraindicated, as lesions typically worsen following trauma in a phenomenon known as "pathergy." The prognosis for patients with PG is generally favorable, though ulcers may recur.

Further reading

1 Weenig RH, Davis MDP, Dahl PR, Su WPD. Skin ulcers misdiagnosed as pyoderma gangrenosum. *New Engl J Med* 2002;**347**(18): 1412–18.
2 Su WP, Davis MD, Weenig RH, Powell FC, Penrry HO. Pyoderma gangrenosum: clinicopathologic correlation and proposed diagnostic criteria. *Int J Dermatol* 2004;**43**(11):790–800.

Case 41 | Chest pain with electrocardiographic ST-segment/T-wave abnormalities

Answer: A
Diagnosis: Left ventricular hypertrophy (LVH)
Discussion: The patient's ECG noted in the case demonstrates a normal sinus rhythm with voltage criteria for left ventricular hypertrophy (S-wave in lead V1 plus the R-wave in lead V6 greater than 35 mm) and ST segment changes (ST segment elevation in leads V1–V3 and ST-segment depression/T-wave inversion in leads I, aVL, V5, and V6). The ST-segment/T-wave changes in this LVH pattern are termed the "strain pattern" (Figure 41.1).

In patients with LVH, ST-segment/T-wave changes are encountered in approximately 70% of cases; these changes result from altered repolarization of the ventricular myocardium due to LVH, representing the "new norm." These

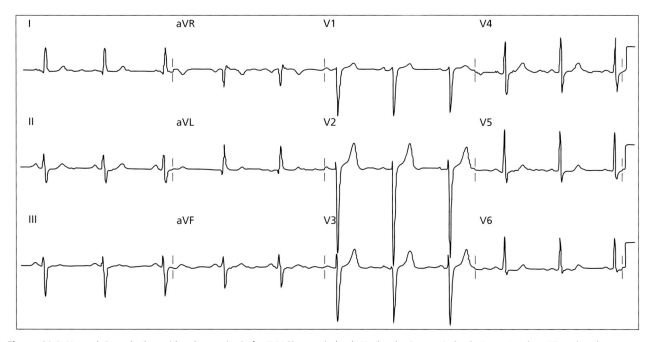

Figure 41.1 Normal sinus rhythm with voltage criteria for LVH (S-wave in lead V1 plus the R-wave in lead V6 greater than 35 mm) and an absence of ST-segment/T-wave abnormalities of significance.

LVH-related ECG changes may mask and/or mimic the early findings consistent with acute coronary ischemia. LVH is associated with poor R-wave progression and loss of the septal R-wave in the right to mid-precordial leads, most commonly producing a QS pattern. In general, these QS complexes are located in leads V1 and V2, rarely extending beyond lead V3. ST segment elevation is encountered in this distribution along with prominent T-waves. The ST segment elevation seen in this distribution is usually 2–4 mm in height though it may reach 5 mm or more – and may be difficult to distinguish from that associated with acute myocardial infarction (AMI). The initial, up-sloping portion of the ST-segment–T-wave complex is frequently concave in LVH compared to the either flattened or convex pattern observed in the patient with AMI.

The "strain" pattern, characterized by downsloping ST segment depression with asymmetric, biphasic, or inverted T-waves in leads with prominent R-waves (the lateral leads I, aVL, V5, and V6) is frequently misinterpreted as acute ischemia. The ST segment/T-wave complex has been described in the following manner: initially bowed upward (convex upward) followed by a gradual downward sloping into an inverted, asymmetrical T-wave with an abrupt return to the baseline. It is important to realize that significant variability may be encountered in the "strain" pattern. The T-wave may be minimally inverted or the inversion may be greater than 5 mm in depth. These T-wave abnormalities may also be encountered in patients lacking prominent voltage (i.e. large S- and R-waves).

Further reading

1 Brady WJ, Lentz B, Barlotta K, Harrigan RA, Chan T. ECG patterns confounding the ECG diagnosis of acute coronary syndrome: left bundle branch block, right ventricular paced rhythms, and left ventricular hypertrophy. *Emerg Med Clin North Am* 2005; **23**(4):999–1025.
2 Somers M, Brady WJ, Perron AD, Mattu A. The prominant T wave: electrocardiographic differential diagnosis. *Am J Emerg Med* 2002;**20**(3):243–51.

Case 42 | **Chemical eye exposure**

Answer: C
Diagnosis: Chemical injury to the eye
Discussion: Chemical injuries to the eye range from mild irritation to devastating destruction of the ocular surface resulting in visual impairment or even loss of the eye. Most chemical injuries affect young patients with exposure occurring at home, in industrial or agricultural accidents, or in criminal assault. The offending chemical may be in the form of a solid, liquid, powder, or vapor. The severity of the injury depends on the offending agent, the surface area of contact, and the degree of penetration.

The most important step in the initial management of chemical injuries is immediate and copious irrigation of the ocular surface with lactated ringers or normal saline solution, even before testing vision. This may be facilitated using a topical anesthetic and handheld intravenous tubing or a Morgan lens. Irrigation should be continued for a minimum of 30 minutes until the conjunctival sac pH is neutral. The conjunctival pH can be easily checked with a urinary pH strip. Sweeping the conjunctival fornices with a moistened cotton-tipped applicator for solid particles should be performed for a persistently elevated pH.

Alkali injuries occur most frequently and are the most devastating. These agents elevate the pH and readily penetrate the ocular tissues. Blanching of the conjunctiva indicates penetration, vascular ischemia, and necrosis which are often the result of severe alkali injuries. On the other hand, acid injuries tend to remain confined to the surface of the eye and produce superficial damage.

Further reading

1 Khah PT, Shah P, Elkington AR. Injury to the eye. *Br Med J* 2004;**328**(7430):36–8.
2 Kuckelkorn R, Schrage N, Keller G, Redbrake C. Emergency treatment of chemical and thermal eye burns. *Acta Ophthalmol Scand* 2002;**80**(1):4–10.

Case 43 | **Hand pain after striking a wall**

Answer: C
Diagnosis: Carpometacarpal (CMC) dislocation of the 4th and 5th metacarpals
Discussion: The CMC joints are extremely stable joints due to significant bony and ligamentous support. As a result, isolated dislocations are not common. Dislocations are usually associated with significant trauma, usually with fractures of the base of the metacarpal. Isolated dislocations do occur, however, and the 4th and 5th are the most common sites since they have the greatest degree of motion and related laxity. CMC dislocations

usually result from extreme forces such as motor vehicle accident, direct blow to the hand, or oblique impact of the closed fist with an immovable object.

The deformity of the dislocated joint is often obscured by the significant soft tissue swelling present on the dorsum of the hand. Tenderness is usually significant. An obvious step-off deformity may be observed and/or palpated at the level of the dislocation (the proximal end of the metacarpal as it over-rides the distal carpus), particularly if the patient presents early prior to the onset of significant swelling. A critical factor in the evaluation is found in the recognition of associated metacarpal fracture. A careful assessment should be made of neurovascular status of the hand. Specific attention should be directed to the status of the deep branch of the ulnar nerve in that it lies immediately volar to the 5th CMC joint; the median nerve may also be injured. Vascular compromise, particularly in patients with injury to the 3rd metacarpal, may involve the deep palmar arterial arch which lies directly beneath the 3rd CMC joint. Integrity of the wrist extensor tendons must be assessed in these dislocation injuries as disruption may occur. Additionally, those patients who have suffered a direct blow are at risk for compartment syndrome in the hand. The anteroposterior radiograph view may reveal an overlap of the carpal bones over the proximal metacarpals (Figure 43.1A, arrow). The lateral radiograph often is diagnostic with obvious dislocation of the CMC joint visualized without problem (Figure 43.1B, arrow).

Treatment in the emergency department consists of closed reduction, which is accomplished with longitudinal traction. The hand should then be splinted; digital motion should be encouraged to prevent stiffness associated with swelling. Orthopedic consultation is necessary as these dislocations often require percutaneous pinning or open reduction with internal fixation.

Further reading

1 Griffiths MA, Moloney DM, Pickford MA. Multiple carpometacarpal dislocations after a low-impact injury: a missed diagnosis. *J Trauma* 2005;**58**:391–2.

2 Kumar S, Arora A, Jain AK, Agarwal A. Volar dislocation of multiple carpometacarpal joints: report of four cases. *J Orthop Trauma* 1998;**12**:523–6.

3 Mabee JR, Lee TJ, Halus S. Dorsal dislocation of the four ulnar metacarpals. *Am J Emerg Med* 1997;**15**:408–11.

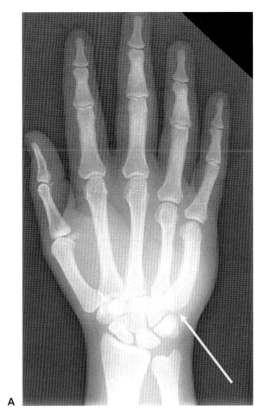

A

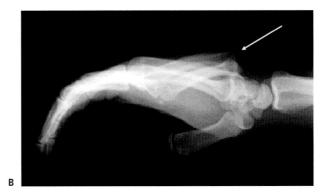

B

Figure 43.1 A Anteroposterior view of the hand and wrist.
B Lateral view of the hand and wrist.

Case 44 | **Dyspnea in an alcoholic**

Answer: E
Diagnosis: Pericardial tamponade
Discussion: Table 44.1 is an overview of the conditions which can be rapidly diagnosed and/or excluded by bedside ultrasound of the thorax and abdomen when confronted by a patient with undifferentiated dyspnea, hypotension, or pulseless electrical activity. Several of these conditions are considerations in the case presented.

Figures 44.1 and 44.2 are images of the heart showing the left ventricle (LV), right ventricle (RV), and a large circumferential pericardial effusion (Figures 44.1 and 44.2; arrows). Effusions are often described as "small/physiological" when they are non-circumferential, "moderate" when they are circumferential but <10 mm in thickness in diastole, large (10–20 mm in thickness), and very large (>20 mm). Although no caliper measurements have been performed, the centimeter markers along the upper margins of the images indicate that this effusion is as large as 40 mm in thickness. Cardiac tamponade is demonstrated in real-time by diastolic collapse of any chamber in the presence of moderate or large effusion. Figure 44.3 shows a right upper quadrant view similar to that used to identify free fluid (FF) in the focused assessment by sonography in trauma (FAST). A very large volume of FF can be seen between the liver and kidney (Morison's pouch). While this could conceivably be blood, its uniformity, complete lack of echogenicity, and marked posterior acoustic enhancement (causing artifactually increased echoes from the underlying tissues marked *), argue against this fluid being intraperitoneal hemorrhage. With the patient's history of alcohol abuse, and the small, hyperechoic liver seen in Figure 44.3, this fluid is much more likely to be due to ascites. In Figure 44.4, a longitudinal view of the upper aorta can be seen showing the celiac and superior mesenteric (SMA) trunks. Probably due to compression, FF is not apparent in this view. Since 90% of abdominal aortic aneurysms (AAA) occur between the renal arteries (1 cm inferior to the SMA) and the bifurcation, aneurysm cannot be excluded based on this view alone. However, there is also no evidence to indicate the presence of AAA.

To summarize, the ultrasound images suggest a variety of abnormalities, which, typical of the resuscitation setting, need to be prioritized according to both their overall likelihood, and potential lethality. The diagnosis that poses the greatest risk of precipitous deterioration is that of cardiac tamponade. It is also the one which would take precedence in management according to the standard emergency medicine priorities of the "ABC's": airway, breathing, and

circulation. Beck's triad is a late finding in tamponade, so that its absence does not exclude the possibility of this diagnosis; which should be made prior to the onset of hypotension. While potentially very serious, intracranial causes of altered mental status are less rapidly lethal than hemodynamic ones, so the latter should be sought and addressed first, especially in a patient with abnormal vital signs such as this one.

With evolving training and experience in bedside sonography, the specialty of emergency medicine has appropriated

Table 44.1 Organs to be investigated and potential diagnoses that may be identified by emergency medicine bedside ultrasound (EMBU) in the evaluation of unexplained hypotension, PEA, or cardiopulmonary arrest.

EMBU of the thorax

Pericardium and heart
Effusion ± tamponade, severe hypovolemia, massive pulmonary embolus, cardiogenic shock, myocardial infarction*, gross valvular dysfunction*
Proximal aorta
Proximal dissection*
Pleural spaces
Pneumothorax, massive pleural effusion, massive pulmonary consolidation

EMBU of the abdomen

Inferior vena cava
Severe hypovolemia, massive pulmonary embolus
Abdominal aorta
Abdominal aortic aneurysm, distal dissection*
Peritoneal cavity
Free fluid, pneumoperitoneum*

*Indicates conditions which can be identified, but cannot be reliably excluded with EMBU.

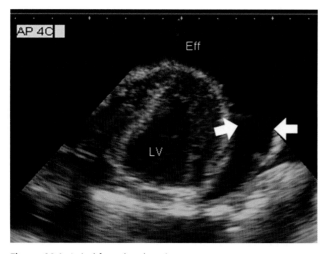

Figure 44.1 Apical four chamber view.

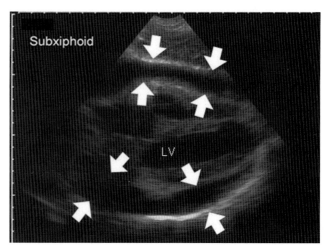

Figure 44.2 Subxiphoid view.

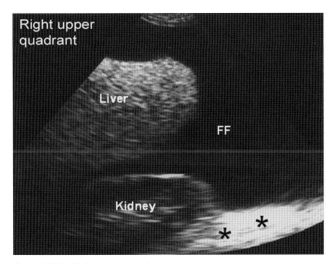

Figure 44.3 Right upper quadrant view.

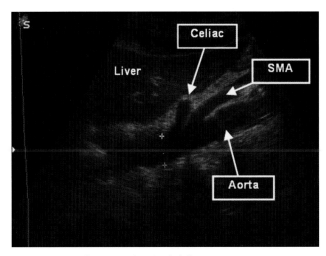

Figure 44.4 Midline sagittal view of abdomen.

and integrated a variety of techniques from disparate specialties to provide rapid information about many of the causes of critical illness. Echocardiographic approaches are used in assessing the heart. Techniques developed in critical care are used to assess the pleural spaces and lungs. The methods of the "FAST" are employed to identify FF in the potential spaces of the abdomen and thorax; and traditional radiological techniques are used to assess the great vessels. In this way, bedside ultrasound performed in real-time by the treating clinician provides immediate diagnostic information about a range of disease processes, many of which mandate therapies that are specific, and mutually exclusive (e.g. volume overload versus hypovolemic shock).

Several algorithms have been proposed to formalize this approach.

Further reading

1 Levine MJ, Lorell BH, Diver DJ, Come PC. Implications of echocardiographically assisted diagnosis of pericardial tamponade in contemporary medical patients: detection before hemodynamic embarrassment. *J Am Coll Cardiol* 1991;**17**(1):59–65.

2 Blaivas M, Graham S, Lambert MJ. Impending cardiac tamponade, an unseen danger? *Am J Emerg Med* 2000;**18**(3):339–40.

3 Rose JS, Bair AE, Mandavia D, Kinser DJ. The UHP ultrasound protocol: a novel ultrasound approach to the empiric evaluation of the undifferentiated hypotensive patient. *Am J Emerg Med* 2001;**19**(4):299–302.

Case 45 | **Slash wound to the neck**

Answer: B

Diagnosis: Zone II neck injury

Discussion: To properly describe a penetrating injury to the neck, it is essential to note the zone of injury, the mechanism of injury, and whether the platysma muscle is violated. Division of the neck into three zones provides clinicians with important anatomic and management information. Zone I (base of the neck) extends from the sternal notch and clavicles to the cricoid cartilage. Zone II (midneck) comprises the area between the cricoid cartilage and the angle of the mandible. Zone III (upper neck) spans the distance between the angle of the mandible and the base of the skull. The platysma muscle is located between the superficial and deep cervical fascia of the

neck. Violation of the platysma muscle should prompt a clinician to suspect injury to the vital structures of the neck.

The treatment of penetrating neck injuries continues to be debated in the surgical literature. Expectant management was the rule prior to World War II and mortality rates were an abysmal 18–35%. In an effort to improve patient survival, a mandatory surgical approach was initiated dropping mortality rates to 6%. This management approach remained the standard of care for decades. However, an increased incidence of negative neck explorations gave rise to the concept of selective surgical management. Selective surgical management aims to reduce the negative neck exploration rate while preserving a low mortality rate for penetrating neck trauma. Under the management scheme of selective surgical exploration, Zone I and Zone III injuries are initially imaged to clearly define a patient's vascular anatomy. Angiography remains the gold standard for diagnosing vascular injuries. The desire for pre-operative imaging stems from the tendency of Zone I injuries to remain clinically concealed and the difficulty associated with surgically approaching Zone III injuries. In contrast, the anatomy of the neck in Zone II is easily approached and explored. Currently, most surgeons choose to surgically explore Zone II injuries without preoperative imaging.

Although the necessity of surgical neck exploration and the reliability of physical examination continue to be debated, serial examinations remain an essential part of the evaluation of a patient with a penetrating neck injury. While unstable patients require immediate airway management (with cervical spine immobilization) and more immediate surgical intervention, stable patients necessitate serial examinations for "soft" and "hard" signs of penetrating neck trauma. Hard signs include expanding hematoma, severe active bleeding, shock not responsive to fluids, decreased or absent radial pulse, vascular bruit or thrill, cerebral ischemia, and airway obstruction. Patients who develop hard signs will likely require surgical intervention. Soft signs include hemoptysis, hematemesis,

dyspnea, dysphonia, dysphagia, subcutaneous or mediastinal air, nonexpanding hematoma, and the presence of focal neurologic deficits.

Patients who are in profound shock or who have uncontrollable hemorrhage from a penetrating neck injury should go directly to the operating room for hemorrhage control. Definitive airway management, large-bore intravenous access and blood samples sent for cross-match are essential in the immediate encounter. Bedside vessel ligation can result in significant neurologic impairment and is not the treatment of choice. Temporary hemorrhage control with direct pressure can be utilized prior to transport to the operating room. An alternative to immediate operative intervention of patients with zone I and zone III injuries depends on the availability of interventional radiology. Angiography and embolization can be utilized in these patients. However, involvement of an interventional radiologist should not delay definitive intervention.

Further reading

1 Thal ER, Meyer DM. Penetrating neck trauma. *Curr Prob Surg* 1992;**29**(1):1–56.
2 McConnell DB, Trunkey DD. Management of penetrating trauma to the neck. *Adv Surg* 1994;**27**:97–127.

Case 46 | **Foot pain following breaking**

Answer: B

Diagnosis: Lisfranc fracture (medial cuneiform and 2nd metatarsal base fracture with lateral displacement of the 2nd–5th metatarsals)

Discussion: The tarsometatarsal joint is named after Jacques Lisfranc, a French physician in Napoleon's army who first described amputations through this joint. Any injury to this joint, from sprain to fracture, is termed a Lisfranc injury. Lisfranc injuries are uncommon because of the high force that is required to disrupt this joint. Lisfranc injuries occur as a result of rotation of the body on a fixed forefoot, axial loading, or crush injuries. Although motor vehicle collisions are usually the mechanism, up to one third of Lisfranc injuries arise from stumbles or falls.

The clinical presentation of a Lisfranc fracture includes severe midfoot pain, inability to bear weight, and paresthesias. Examination often reveals edema, ecchymosis, and midfoot tenderness. Patients with severe injuries may have obvious deformity of the midfoot with forefoot displacement. Vascular injury may occur because a branch of the dorsalis pedis artery dives between the 1st and 2nd metatarsal, forming the plantar arch. Injury to this vessel is uncommon, however, and can

lead to hemorrhage, vascular compromise, and compartment syndrome. Radiographic findings suggestive of a Lisfranc injury include widening between the 1st and 2nd or 2nd and 3rd metatarsal base. In addition, any fracture involving the Lisfranc joint (base of the metatarsals, cuboid, and cuneiforms) should raise suspicion for joint disruption. A fracture involving the 2nd metatarsal base is virtually pathognomonic for Lisfranc joint injury.

Management of a Lisfranc fracture is operative and requires an orthopedic consultation. The patient requires serial vascular checks, however, doesn't need an angiogram without evidence of vascular compromise. Although rapid reduction of the displaced metatarsals is desirable, the patient does not require emergent reduction, as the fracture does not compromise skin or vascular structures.

Further reading

1 Perron AD, Brady WJ. Evaluation and management of the high-risk orthopedic emergency. *Emerg Med Clin North Am* 2003; **21**(1):159–204.
2 Perron AD, Brady WJ, Keats TE. Orthopedic pitfalls in the ED: Lisfranc fracture-dislocation. *Am J Emerg Med* 2001;**19**(1):71–5.

Case 47 | **Confluent rash in a child**

Answer: C

Diagnosis: Erythema multiforme (minor)

Discussion: Erythema multiforme (EM) is a hypersensitivity reaction which manifests as a diffuse eruption with very characteristic lesions. These lesions are usually symmetric, involve palms of hands and soles of feet, and predominate on the extensor surfaces of the upper and lower extremities. Although these are characteristic locations they can be found anywhere on the body. The rash of EM can look macular, urticarial, or vesicobullous, but the prototypical lesion is a target lesion with a dusky center. Often the rash changes from one form of lesion to another as the disease progresses. The rash itself generally lasts at least 1 week, but can last up to 6 weeks. Patients are often otherwise asymptomatic although they can also have itching associated with the lesions or involvement of the oral mucosa.

The causes of EM are often unknown, but in children are most commonly related to infectious causes, whereas in adults it is much more frequently related to drug reaction or malignancy. The most common infectious agent attributed to EM is herpes simplex virus. The differential diagnosis of EM includes pemphigus, bullous pemphigoid, urticaria, or other viral exanthema. Treatment for EM minor may involve cessation of inciting agents, but is mainly supportive including antihistamines and/or NSAIDS. Systemic glucocorticoids are sometimes used although there are no randomized trials showing a clear benefit.

It is important to note that EM is thought to be part of continuum of more serious illness such as Stevens–Johnson (EM major) and toxic epidermal necrolysis (TEN). It is important on physical exam to evaluate mucosal surfaces to differentiate between EM minor and major. EM minor involves the skin and only one other mucosal surface, usually the mouth. In contrast, Stevens–Johnson involves the eye, oral cavity, genital mucosa, upper airway, or esophagus. Stevens–Johnson and TEN are much more serious conditions with significantly higher mortality rates. Treatment for these conditions is frequently compared to burn care and hospital admission is required. It is important to keep these other entities in mind even in cases of EM minor because patients and their families should be discharged with clear instructions about signs to look for that may indicate progression to more serious disease.

Further reading

1 Carder KR. Hypersensitivity reactions in neonates and infants. *Dermatol Ther* 2005;**18**(2):160–75.
2 William PM, Konklin RJ. Erythema multiforme: a review and contrast from Stevens-Johnson syndrome/toxic epidermal necrolysis. *Dent Clin North Am* 2005;**49**(1): 67–76.

Case 48 | **Lost in the cold**

Answer: B

Diagnosis: Frostbite

Discussion: Frostbite is a cold-related injury that is due to the freezing of tissues when exposed to temperatures at or below the freezing point of intact skin. As the temperature to the skin drops, blood flow diminishes, ice crystals form, osmotic disequilibrium occurs, cellular dehydration develops, and cellular wall integrity becomes compromised. The end result is cellular death and capillary damage.

Initial management should first be directed at assessing core body temperature and hydration. Both active and passive rewarming may be considered, depending on the patient's core body temperature. Most patients will also benefit from intravenous fluid administration as some degree of dehydration is typically seen.

After initial stabilization, rapid rewarming of the afflicted extremity is of paramount importance. A warm water bath at temperatures between 40°C and 42°C is the recommended for approximately 30 minutes. Utilizing water at lower temperatures results in slower and potentially incomplete rewarming which worsens outcome; utilizing water at higher temperatures risks the development of thermal burns. As extremity reperfusion begins, severe pain can be expected and opioid analgesics are typically required. Dry air rewarming, especially over a campfire, is discouraged because of the possibility of thermal injury. Massaging the frostbitten extremity should be avoided as it may result in further tissue damage.

After rewarming, attention is directed toward wound care and pain control. Wounds should be wrapped in sterile gauze after application of topical Aloe vera. Aloe vera is an inhibitor of thromboxane which is thought to play a large role in tissue loss. Ibuprofen should also be given because of its ability to inhibit thromboxane. Tetanus immunization status should be assessed and the patient should avoid smoking.

Considerable controversy exists in regard to management of blisters. Clear vesicles and bullae are rich in thromboxane, which is thought to increase tissue loss. Aspiration of these bullae has been advocated as a way to remove the immune modulators while preserving the barrier to infections. Others have advocated debridement as a means to remove thromboxane and allow for direct application of Aloe vera.

Surgical management of frostbite injuries should be delayed. There are three zones of injury: (1) the distal zone which progresses to dry gangrene and eventually requires amputation; (2) the proximal zone which heals without intervention; (3) the intermediate zone which has the potential for salvage. Treatment and wound care are directed toward this zone in hope of salvaging as much tissue as possible. Complications may occur that require surgical intervention (i.e. compartment syndrome or gas gangrene), but the available evidence does not suggest that early debridement of afflicted tissue improves outcome.

Heparin therapy has been shown to be of benefit in some animal models. Thrombosis of the microvasculature is a frequent finding after rewarming and may contribute to tissue loss. Heparin therapy was directed at reversing this thrombosis. Currently available human studies, however, have failed to show any benefit of heparin therapy over rapid rewarming and general wound care.

Further reading

1 Biem J, Koehncke N, Classen D, Dosman J. Out of the cold: management of hypothermia and frostbite. *Can Med Assoc J* 2003;**168**(3):305–11.
2 Murphy JV, Banwell PE, Roberts AH, McGrouther DA. Frostbite: pathogenesis and treatment. *J Trauma* 2000;**48**(1):171–8.
3 Reamy BV. Frostbite: review and current concepts. *J Am Board Fam Pract* 1998;**11**(1):34–40.

Case 49 | **Bradycardia following an herbal ingestion**

Answer: E

Diagnosis: *Aconitum dephinifolium* (monkshood) poisoning

Discussion: The use of herbal products has dramatically increased over the past decade, driving physicians to become educated in regards to potential herbal complications and drug interactions. Studies have documented that approximately one in every five patients presenting to the emergency department uses some type of herbal preparation.

Plants that contain aconitine include *Aconitum napellus* (monkshood), *A. vulparia* (wolfsbane), *A. carmichaeli* (chuanwu), and *A. kusnezoffii* (caowu). Members of this plant genus grow throughout the world. Aconitine exposures are commonly associated with the overzealous consumption of certain herbal preparations. Although a number of fatal poisonings have been reported, aconitine is still readily available at many nutrition or herbal medicine stores.

These flowers of the plant, which are commonly purple, form a hood-like structure, hence the name "monkshood." All parts of this plant are potentially poisonous. Aconitine appears to increase sodium entry into muscle, nerve, baroreceptors, and Purkinje fibers to produce a positive inotropic effect, enhanced vagal tone, neurotoxicity, increased automaticity, and torsade de pointe. Bifascicular ventricular tachycardia, a

dysrhythmia most frequently associated with digitalis toxicity, has also been reported in patients poisoned with aconitine.

Following exposure, symptoms have been reported to occur between 3 minutes and 2 hours, with a median of 30 minutes. Symptoms may persist for up to 30 hours. Neurologic complaints include initial visual impairment, dizziness, limb paresthesias, weakness, ataxia, and coma. Chest discomfort, dyspnea, tachycardia, bradycardia, ectopic beats, supraventricular tachycardia, bundle branch block, intermittent bigeminy, ventricular tachycardia, ventricular fibrillation, and asystole have all been described.

Treatment is primarily supportive. The paramount concern is management of lethal arrhythmias. Symptomatic bradydysrhythmias may respond to atropine administration. Ventricular tachycardia has been reported to be refractory to pharmacologic therapy.

Further reading

1 Guha S, Dawn B, Dutta G, *et al.* Bradycardia, reversible panconduction defect and syncope following self-medication with a homeopathic medicine. *Cardiology* 1999;**91**(4):268–71.
2 Furbee B, Wermuth M. Life-threatening plant poisoning. *Crit Care Clin* 1997;**13**(4):849–88.

Case 50 | **Abdominal pain in an alcoholic**

Answer: C

Diagnosis: Sentinel loop

Discussion: The term *sentinel loop* was first used in 1946 by Levitin. On plain film, he described it as an isolated loop of distended adynamic bowel. A sentinel loop may be seen on radiograph when there is localized inflammation in the peritoneal cavity. A segmental paralytic ileus affecting one or two loops of small bowel may subsequently occur adjacent to this localized inflammation. Gas and fluid accumulate in this isolated area of small bowel as the localized inflammatory process leads to a focal decrease in peristalsis.

There are various disease processes that may lead to a sentinel loop on radiograph. When found in the upper abdomen, a sentinel loop may be due to pancreatitis, cholecystitis, or less commonly pyelonephritis or splenic injury. In acute pancreatitis, while many various radiographic findings may appear on plain film, the sentinel loop is the most specific. Appendicitis may lead to a sentinel loop on plain film in the right lower quadrant. The sentinel loop is a nonspecific radiographic finding and sometimes may mimic small or even large bowel obstruction.

Further reading

1 Davis S, Parbhoo SP, Gibson MJ. The plain abdominal radiograph in acute pancreatitis. *Clin Radiol* 1980;**31**(1): 87–93.
2 Ranson JH. Diagnostic standards for acute pancreatitis. *World J Surg* 1997;**21**(2):136–42.

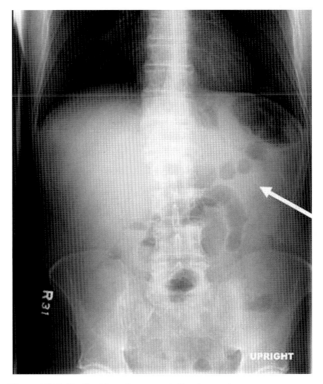

Figure 50.1 Sentinel loop (arrow pointing to area).

Case 51 | **Pain out of proportion to examination**

Answer: E

Diagnosis: Clostridial myonecrosis (gas gangrene)

Discussion: Clostridial myonecrosis, which is more commonly known as gas gangrene, is a surgical emergency. *Clostridium perfringens* is the most common pathogen isolated, but many clostridial species are capable of producing the disease. Exotoxins, which are produced under anerobic conditions, are responsible for morbidity and mortality associated with clostridial myonecrosis. These toxins result in numerous detrimental effects, including lysis of muscle cells, destruction of blood vessels, hemolysis, and cardiac suppression.

The clinical picture can initially appear benign, necessitating vigilance in making this clinical diagnosis. Pain is rapidly progressive over hours to days and is typically out of proportion to physical findings. Low-grade fever is common and is lower than would be expected given the severity of the infection. The wound itself is usually unimpressive with surrounding pale tissue. In later stages the wound can appear dusky and progress to dark discoloration. Wound discharge is commonly foul-smelling and brown, with a blood tinged appearance. This wound discharge should be sent for culture and Gram stain, and typically reveals a preponderance of Gram-positive rods and a lack of neutrophils. Gas in the soft tissues can clinically manifest as crepitus. Radiographic evidence of air in the soft tissues suggests the diagnosis (as noted in the X-ray of this case). Some authors advocate sonography as a tool to identify gas in the wound before it is apparent clinically or on plain radiographs.

Once the diagnosis is entertained, empiric therapy should be initiated immediately. Intravenous penicillin should be given in doses of 12–16 million international units per day divided in four daily doses. Emergent surgical evaluation is essential. Usually multiple surgeries are needed to ensure adequate debridement. Radical excision and amputation are commonly necessary to prevent mortality (as occurred in this case). Aggressive fluid resuscitation should be initiated in the emergency department as hypotension and septic shock are commonly encountered. Hyperbaric oxygen therapy has been advocated as an adjunctive modality, but must be used in concert with intravenous antibiotics and surgical debridement.

Further reading

1 Gonzalez MH. Necrotizing fasciitis and gangrene of the upper extremity. *Hand Clin* 1998;**14**(4):635–45.
2 Headley AJ. Necrotizing soft tissue infections: a primary care review. *Am Fam Physician* 2003;**68**(2):323–8.

Case 52 | **Pleuritic chest pain in a young adult male**

Answer: D

Diagnosis: Acute pericarditis

Discussion: The ECG is typical of acute myopericarditis with pericardial effusion manifested by electrical alternans. The rhythm strip demonstrates electrical alternans with alternating QRS complex amplitudes. The ECG demonstrates significant, diffuse ST segment elevation with a concave morphology; additionally, PR segment depression is seen in most leads with ST segment elevation. Lead aVr demonstrates reciprocal PR segment elevation.

Acute pericarditis produces diffuse inflammation of the pericardium and superficial epicardium. Numerous etiologies are encountered in the patient with acute myopericarditis, including infectious, inflammatory, toxicologic, and rheumatologic causes. The ECG can demonstrate significant findings in patients with acute pericarditis, including ST segment elevation, T-wave inversion, and PR segment abnormalities. These changes result from endocardial inflammation; it is important to realize that the pericardium is electrically silent. Because of involvement of the pericardium and endocardium, pericarditis is most appropriately termed *myopericarditis*.

The ECG changes caused by pericarditis evolve through four classic stages. The first stage is characterized by ST segment elevation which is followed by resolution of the elevation in the second stage. The third stage occurs with T-wave inversion followed by normalization of all such changes and a return to the baseline ECG in stage four. The temporal evolution of these electrocardiographic stages occurs in a very unpredictable fashion – stages one through three are seen over hours to days while stage four may not be reached for several weeks. Further, patients may not manifest all characteristic ECG features.

ST segment elevation seen in patients with stage one pericarditis is usually less than 5 mm in height, observed in numerous leads, and characterized by a concavity to its initial upsloping portion. The ST segment elevation is most often seen in multiple leads though it may be limited to a specific anatomic segment. PR segment depression associated with pericarditis perhaps is the most helpful feature in arriving at the correct electrocardiographic diagnosis; such a finding has been described as "almost diagnostic" for acute pericarditis. Reciprocal PR segment elevation is seen in lead aVr and is usually very helpful in the diagnosis.

Pericardial effusion may also be seen in patients with pericarditis; the presence of the effusion may affect the electrocardiographic signal noted on the ECG. These findings include widespread low voltage (resulting from increased resistance to injury current flow with the accumulated fluid) and electrical alternans (a beat-to-beat alteration in QRS complex size due to shifting fluid in the pericardium).

Further reading

1 Chan T, Brady WJ, Pollack M. Electrocardiographic manifestations: acute myopericarditis. *J Emerg Med* 1999;**17**:865–72.
2 Lange RA, Hillis LD. Clinical practice: acute pericarditis. *New Engl J Med* 2004;**351**(21):2195–202.

Case 53 | **Eye pain following a bar fight**

Answer: D

Diagnosis: Full thickness lid laceration

Discussion: This patient has two full thickness lid lacerations to the left lower lid. When a patient presents with an apparent isolated lid laceration, it is necessary to first exclude globe injury or rupture. Determining the mechanism of injury with a thorough history will help direct management. Complete ocular examination is necessary to rule out globe injury. Examination should include visual acuity, pupils, extraocular motility, external adnexa, slit lamp examination, tonometry, and dilated fundus exam. Computed tomography scan of the brain and orbit (axial and coronal views), using 1–3 mm cuts, should be obtained when a foreign body or globe rupture is suspected. Tetanus prophylaxis should be given when indicated.

The presence of fat in a periocular wound indicates that the orbital septum has been violated. In these cases it is necessary to determine if damage to the levator muscle has occurred. Lacerations occurring in the medial canthal area require evaluation of the lacrimal drainage system.

Many eyelid lacerations can be repaired in the emergency room. Lid lacerations requiring repair in the operating room include those involving the lacrimal drainage apparatus, involvement of the levator muscle, extensive tissue loss, or associated globe trauma requiring surgery.

Further reading

1 Chang EL, Rubin PA. Management of complex eyelid lacerations. *Int Ophthalmol Clin* 2002;**42**(3):187–201.
2 Larian B, Wong B, Crumley RL, *et al.* Facial trauma and ocular/orbital injury. *J Craniomaxillofac Trauma* 1999;**5**(4):15–24.

Case 54 | **Forearm fracture after falling**

Answer: E

Diagnosis: Monteggia fracture

Discussion: A Monteggia fracture is an eponym for an ulnar fracture associated with a dislocation of the radial head. The dislocation of the radial head (note how the line along the axis of the radius does not intersect the capitellum in Figure 54.1) can be easily overlooked if the radiographs fail to include the elbow. If the radial head dislocation is missed, prolonged disarticulation and subsequent disability may occur. Monteggia fractures can result from falling on an outstretched hand with forced pronation. The energy exerted in fracturing the ulna travels along the interosseus membrane pulling the radial head from the annular ligament.

Reduction of the radial head must be achieved expeditiously followed by splinting of the forearm in a position of function with wrist extended. Monteggia fractures are often managed with internal fixation because of the increased risk of non-union.

Radial motor nerve injury can occur from stretching or compressing the nerve as it passes across the elbow. The radial nerve becomes the posterior interosseous nerve which supplies the extensor muscles of the wrist, fingers, and thumb. Motor neuropathies are usually treated with conservative management with surgical exploration being reserved for those who do not regain function within 2–3 months.

A Galeazzi fracture is an eponym for a radial fracture associated with the dislocation of the distal radioulnar joint. Galeazzi fractures are typically treated with open reduction and internal fixation.

Further reading

1 Wilkins KE. Changes in the management of Monteggia fractures. *J Pediatr Orthop* 2002;**22**(4):548–54.
2 Perron AD, Hersh RE, Brady WJ, Keats TE. Orthopedic pitfalls in the ED: Galeazzi and Monteggia fracture–dislocation. *Am J Emerg Med* 2001;**19**(3):225–8.

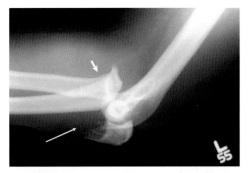

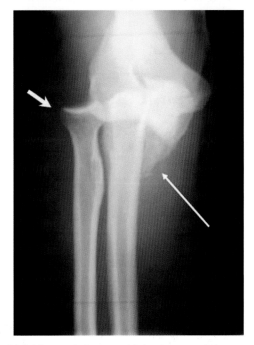

Figure 54.1 Monteggia fracture with long arrow pointing to proximal ulnar fracture and short arrow pointing to radial head dislocation.

Case 55 | An elderly woman with groin pain

Answer: B
Diagnosis: Avascular necrosis (AVN) of the left femoral head
Discussion: Patients presenting with progressive groin and/or thigh pain radiating to the buttock must be evaluated for AVN of the femoral head. AVN is a progressive disease of joint destruction with many causes. Steroid exposure, alcoholism, hemoglobinopathies, renal disease, and a history of hip fracture or hip dislocation all put patients at risk for ischemia of the femoral head. Independent of the precipitating event, all patients with ischemic bone soon develop abnormal bone growth, edema, and fibrosis. Males are at higher risk for AVN and it typically develops in patients after the age of 40 years. Groin pain that is worse with weight bearing and limited range of motion of the affected joint are common initial complaints. Plain radiographic findings can lag behind clinical symptoms of hip pain and difficulty walking.

Diagnosis is dependent upon clinical suspicion and confirmed by radiographic studies. The plain radiographic studies to obtain include anteroposterior and frog leg lateral views (frog leg views allow for evaluation of the superior portion of the femoral head). A staging system exists for AVN. In stage one, plain radiographs are normal but if the clinician has a high index of suspicion diagnosis can be achieved using magnetic resonance imaging. Stage two is characterized by diffuse osteoporosis of the femoral head; therefore subchondral lytic lesions can be seen on plain radiography but the shape of the femoral head is preserved. In the third stage, many of the pathognomonic changes become evident on radiography; there is frank collapse of bone, the crescent sign may be seen (subchondral radiolucency), and there is flattening of the femoral head. The fourth stage is progression of subchondral bone collapse including marked deformity of the femoral head with or without acetabular involvement. In comparison to osteoarthritis, the joint space is preserved until late in the disease process when the entire joint has collapsed.

A clinical syndrome of AVN also has a staging system, but it has not been demonstrated to correlate well with the X-ray findings or disease progression. Treatment for AVN initially includes avoidance of weight bearing if caught early, but this disease typically progresses to the need for joint replacement.

Further reading
1 Musso ES, Mitchell SN, Schink-Ascani M, Bassett CA. Results of conservative management of osteonecrosis of the femoral head: a retrospective review. *Clin Orthop Relat Res* 1986;(207):209–15.
2 Mont MA, Payman RK, Laporte DM, *et al.* Atraumatic osteonecrosis of the humeral head. *J Rheumatol* 2000;**27**(7):1766–73.

Case 56 | Painful facial rash

Answer: E
Diagnosis: Herpes zoster ophthalmicus
Discussion: Herpes zoster ophthalmicus is a reactivation of the varicella virus affecting the ophthalmic division of the trigeminal nerve. It is important to perform a careful medical history on patients presenting with herpes zoster ophthalmicus to determine whether the patient may be immunocompromised. Patients younger than 40 years require a complete systemic evaluation. Older patients do not require evaluation unless immunodeficiency is suspected from the case history.

Ocular manifestations of herpes zoster ophthalmicus are immense and often require long-term follow-up. When herpes zoster ophthalmicus affects the tip of the nose this is known as Hutchinson's sign, indicating involvement of the nasociliary branch of the ophthalmic division. There is a higher risk of ocular involvement in patients with a positive Hutchinson's sign. Ocular evaluation for patients with herpes zoster ophthalmicus includes visual acuity, intraocular pressures, careful slit lamp examination, and a dilated fundus exam.

Patients with active skin lesions for less than 72 hours should be started on an oral antiviral agent such as acyclovir, 800 mg five times a day or famciclovir, 500 mg three times a day. Patients that are systemically ill or immunocompromised should be admitted to the hospital and given intravenous acyclovir. Bacitracin or erythromycin ointment should be applied to the skin lesions three times a day. Patients with ocular involvement need ophthalmologic consultation since they may require corticosteroid therapy and regular outpatient follow-up. A primary physician should also manage these patients since pain from herpes zoster ophthalmicus is often severe and post-herpetic neuralgia can linger for months.

Further reading
1 Baran R, Kechijian P. Hutchinson's sign: a reappraisal. *J Am Acad Dermatol* 1996;**34**(1):87–90.
2 Yoshida M, Hayasaka S, Yamada T, *et al.* Ocular findings in Japanese patients with varicella-zoster virus infection. *Ophthalmologica* 2005;**219**(5):272–5.

Case 57 | Confusion, anemia, and abdominal pain in a toddler

Answer: D

Diagnosis: Lead encephalopathy due to ingestion of paint chips

Discussion: There are multiple radioopacities noted in the plain film consistent with ingestion of paint chips (Figure 57.1).

A list of the more common radioopacities is summarized by the mnemonic CHIPES – calcium/chloral hydrate, heavy metals/halogenated hydrocarbons, iron, phenothiazines/potassium, enteric-coated, and salicylates. However, multiple studies regarding the radioopacity of ingested pharmaceuticals have not consistently supported this and other mnemonics.

A federal mandate banned the use of lead in house and furniture paint since 1978. Any child who lives or has contact with houses built before this time is at risk for elevated lead levels through ingestion of chips or by frequent hand-to-mouth activity in the dust-laden dilapidated environment. Children have fairly efficient absorption of lead, averaging 40–50%. Lead affects multiple organ systems by disrupting various enzymatic activities. In children, subtle clinical effects may be seen even at low lead levels (<10 μg/dL). Obvious acute neurotoxicity at much higher levels is attributable to cerebral edema from fluid egress across the blood–brain barrier. Lead disrupts many of the enzymes in heme biosynthesis resulting in a microcytic hypochromic anemia that mimics iron deficiency anemia. Vomiting, anorexia, constipation, and "lead colic" have all been described in children.

Lead encephalopathy, as demonstrated in this case, must be treated emergently with chelation therapy. British antilewisite (BAL) is the chelator of choice because it readily crosses the blood–brain barrier. BAL is the only chelator that is both renally cleared and biliarly cleared. The disadvantages to BAL include the following: (1) it is administered only by intramuscular injection; (2) it is exceedingly painful and needs to be mixed with an anesthetic such as procaine; (3) it is mixed in peanut oil and cannot be given to children with known peanut allergies. Calcium disodium ethylenediaminetetraacetate (CaNa2EDTA), the only other parenteral chelator, does

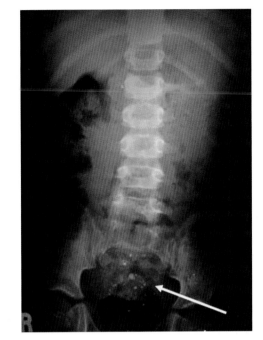

Figure 57.1 Ingestion of paint chips.

not cross the blood–brain barrier. Administration of CaNa2EDTA solely without BAL could place the patient at risk for progressive cerebral edema by mobilizing lead from the other tissues and causing it to redistribute into the brain.

Asymptomatic children should be chelated with oral 2,3-dimercaptosuccinic acid (DMSA) at levels only exceeding 44 μg/dL. Health Department notification should be made at blood lead levels at or exceeding 10 μg/dL.

Further reading

1 Gordon RA, Roberts G, Amim Z, Williams RH, Paloucek FP. Aggressive approach in the treatment of acute lead encephalopathy with an extraordinarily high concentration of lead. *Arch Pediatr Adolesc Med* 1998;**152**(11):1100–04.

2 Feldman RG, White RF. Lead neurotoxicity and disorders of learning. *J Child Neurol* 1992;**7**(4):354–9.

Case 58 | Cardiotoxic effects following caustic ingestion

Answer: B

Diagnosis: Fluoride toxicity

Discussion: In this case, the patient ingested an unknown liquid substance. His initial symptoms of throat burning, emesis, difficulty with phonation, inability to manage secretions, and chest and abdominal pain were consistent with a caustic

ingestion. A rapid bedside litmus paper test revealed that the substance had an acidic pH. An initial arterial blood gas revealed a metabolic acidosis with concomitant respiratory alkalosis. The patient subsequently progressed to hypotension with electrocardiographic (ECG) changes of both QRS complex widening and QT interval prolongation. For the astute clinician who considers the differential diagnosis for an acidic agent that produces metabolic acidosis, hypotension, and ECG abnormalities (QRS complex widening and QT interval prolongation), the diagnosis is readily determined to be hydrofluoric acid ingestion.

Hydrofluoric acid is utilized in many industrial settings for the production of integrated circuits, fluorides, plastics, germicides, insecticides and for the etching and cleaning of silicone, glass, metal, stone, and porcelain. Hydrofluoric acid containing products are sold as automotive cleaning products in local stores. Hydrofluoric acid rapidly corrodes and penetrates skin and mucous membranes. Ingestion of hydrofluoric acid may result in local mucosal caustic effects, nausea, vomiting, abdominal pain, and hemorrhagic gastritis. Systemic electrolyte abnormalities may occur. The absorbed fluoride ions rapidly bind to available calcium and magnesium ions, decreasing the body's levels of these divalent cations. Hyperkalemia often follows due to an efflux of potassium out of cells into the extracellular space.

This patient manifested progressive QT interval prolongation. Hydrofluoric acid causes QT interval prolongation by inducing hypomagnesemia and hypocalcemia. These events may place the patient at risk for polymorphic ventricular tachycardia or torsades de pointes.

All patients presenting with signs and symptoms consistent with hydrofluoric acid ingestion should be aggressively managed. The patient's airway should be patent and adequate ventilation assured. If necessary, endotracheal tube intubation should be performed early before edema leads to airway obstruction. The patient should be placed on continuous cardiac monitoring with pulse oximetry and frequent neurological checks should be made. The initial treatment of hypotension consists of intravenous fluids, followed by pressors as needed. The patient's pulmonary status should be monitored closely for clinical signs consistent with pulmonary aspiration. Activated charcoal, syrup of ipecac, and gastric lavage are absolutely contraindicated in patients who have ingested caustics. Serum electrolytes should be obtained hourly and include serial calcium, magnesium, and potassium levels. The clinician should obtain serial ECGs looking for signs of hypocalcemia (prolonged QTc interval) and hyperkalemia (peaked T-waves). Large amounts of calcium and magnesium may be needed to normalize serum levels. Fluoride-induced hyperkalemia has been reported to be difficult to reverse. Early aggressive therapy with glucose, insulin and/or sodium bicarbonate may be effective.

Dermal hydrofluoric acid exposures are more commonly seen than ingestions and occur when household rust removers or tire cleaners are used (concentrations range from 6% to 12%). These agents often cause delayed finger pain after liquid drips from the spray bottle onto unprotected hands during application of the product. The exposed dermal site may initially look quite innocuous and still cause significant local and potentially systemic toxicity. Inhalational exposures can cause laryngeal, pharyngeal, or pulmonary edema. Ocular exposure can lead to extensive damage to the eye similar to other acids with copious irrigation as the mainstay of treatment.

Symptomatic hand exposures can be treated with topical gels (25 mL of 10% calcium gluconate in 75 mL of a water-soluble lubricant such a KY Jelly). In cases with refractory pain, some authors have advised arterial catheter placement proximal (radial artery) in the exposed hand and infusion of calcium gluconate. A typical infusion regimen is as follows: a 10 mL solution of calcium gluconate mixed in 50 mL of 5% dextrose in water and infused over 4 hours.

Further reading

1 Holstege CP, Baer AB, Brady WJ. The electrocardiographic toxidrome: the ECG presentation of hydrofluoric acid ingestion. *Am J Emerg Med* 2005;**23**:171–6.
2 Bertolini JC. Hydrofluoric acid: a review of toxicity. *J Emerg Med* 1992;**10**(2):163–8.

Case 59 | **Rash and joint pain in a child**

Answer: A

Diagnosis: Henoch–Schönlein purpura (HSP)

Discussion: HSP is the most common systemic vasculitis in children, with rapid onset over the course of days to weeks. The disease is an example of a leukocytoclastic vasculitis, characterized by immune complex deposition leading to necrosis and inflammation of small blood vessels, most commonly the postcapillary venules. The disease course is usually over 6 weeks, with the majority of patients resolving their disease in 1 month. Relapses can occur in 16–40% of patients, up to 2 years after the initial symptoms. Clinical manifestations of HSP are seen in several organ systems including the skin, joints, gastrointestinal tract, and kidney.

Cutaneous involvement is seen in 100% of patients and is characterized by palpable purpura, most commonly on the lower extremities and in dependent areas, such as the posterior thighs and buttocks. However, the rash can involve upper extremities as well. When the rash is more widespread, it is imperative to differentiate HSP from more serious conditions such as meningococcemia, idiopathic thrombocytopenic purpura (ITP), subacute bacterial endocarditis (SBE) and hemolytic uremic syndrome (HUS).

Joint involvement occurs in 50–80% of patients with HSP, and commonly involves large lower extremity joints, such as knees and ankles. True arthritis is rare, but pain, periarticular swelling and limitation of range of motion can be significant. Usually anti-inflammatory medications such as naproxen or Ibuprofen are helpful for these symptoms. Arthrocentesis is not indicated.

Gastrointestinal involvement is seen in 65–70% of patients with HSP, usually within 1–4 weeks of the onset of rash. Rarely (14–36%) patients may have abdominal pain before the rash is evident. The symptoms usually involve colicky periumbilical pain and vomiting, with or without abdominal distention. This results from submucosal and subserosal edema and hemorrhage. Rarely, emergent gastrointestinal complications such as small bowel intussusception, bowel ischemia and infarction, and bowel perforation may occur. Although no evidence in the literature supports the use of glucocorticoids for treatment of abdominal pain, traditionally they are used in hope of shortening the duration of the gastrointestinal symptoms. Steroids have no effect on the overall course of the disease.

The most significant morbidity associated with HSP is secondary to renal involvement. It is the risk of renal involvement which will dictate the close follow-up these patients require. Renal disease can occur in 20–34% of patients with HSP, and the spectrum ranges from microscopic hematuria, with or without proteinuria, to fulminant renal failure which can occur in 1–5% of patients. Due to this small yet significant risk, patients with HSP need weekly blood pressure checks and weekly urinalyses throughout the course of disease.

Overall, HSP is a benign vasculitic disease of childhood, requiring mostly supportive care. Two-thirds of patients will resolve their symptoms within 1 month of onset. Close follow-up by a primary care physician is appropriate for the majority of cases.

Further reading

1 Lanzkowsky S, Lanzkowsky L, Lanzkowsky P. Henoch–Schoenlein purpura. *Pediatr Rev* 1992;**13**(4):130–7.
2 Saulsbury FT. Henoch–Schonlein purpura in children. Report of 100 patients and review of the literature. *Medicine* 1999;**78**(6):395–409.

Case 60 | X-ray findings after laparoscopy

Answer: B

Diagnosis: Post-operative pneumoperitoneum

Discussion: Pneumoperitoneum refers to air within the peritoneal cavity. It characteristically appears as radiolucency between the right hemi-diaphragm and the liver, or in a superiorly dependent location on abdominal radiograph. It usually indicates a perforated abdominal viscus. Tumor, ulcers, or trauma may cause any portion of the bowel to perforate, leading to an associated peritonitis that typically requires urgent abdominal surgery. Pneumoperitoneum does not require surgery in 5–15% cases.

Nonsurgical pneumoperitoneum (NSP) is defined by the presence of air in the peritoneal space that is detectable by plain film X-rays and either is managed successfully by observation and supportive care alone or results in a nondiagnostic laparotomy. NSP is most commonly retained post-operative air. It may occur after peritoneal dialysis catheter placement, gastrointestinal endoscopic procedures, mechanical ventilation, cardiopulmonary resuscitation, pneumothorax, pneumomediastinum, sexual intercourse, or vaginal douching.

Post-operative pneumoperitoneum usually resolves 3–6 days after surgery, although it may persist for as long as 24 days. When abdominal pain and distention are minimal, and peritoneal signs and evidence of a systemic inflammatory response (fever, tachycardia, leukocytosis, and tachypnea) are absent, conservative management is appropriate.

Further reading

1 Mularski RA, Sippel JM, Osborne ML. Pneumoperitoneum: a review of nonsurgical causes. *Crit Care Med* 2000;**28**(7):2638–44.
2 Roberts PA, Wrenn K, Lundquist S. Pneumoperitoneum after percutaneous endoscopic gastrostomy: a case report and review. *J Emerg Med* 2005;**28**(1):45–8.
3 Rosen DM, Lam AM, Chapman M, Carlton M, Cario GM. Methods of creating pneumoperitoneum: a review of techniques and complications. *Obstet Gynecol Surv* 1998;**53**(3):167–74.

Case 61 | Injector injury to the hand

Answer: D

Diagnosis: High-pressure injection injury

Discussion: Injection injuries that involve the hand and/or upper extremity are uncommon and most are job related.

The advent of high-pressure industrial equipment has led to the occurrence of injection of fuel oil, grease, cement, paints, and solvents in the body. The lower the viscosity of the injected substance the higher the potential for spread through

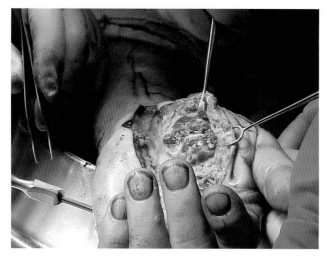

Figure 61.1 Surgical exploration of the case noted above. Note the marked tissue edema and damage induced.

soft tissue. A pressure of 100 pounds per square inch (psi) can breach the skin. It is not uncommon for airless spray-guns or fuel injectors to generate 3000–5000 psi.

The patient who presents with this type of injury is typically a young male who has injured his non-dominant hand. The injured site commonly appears as a small harmless puncture

with some surrounding soft tissue swelling. Clinicians should not be misled by this innocuous presentation as significant functional morbidity and loss of limb are possible.

Emergent management should include tetanus prophy-laxis, analgesia, and broad-spectrum antibiotics. Radiographs of the involved areas can help determine the extent of the soft tissue spread of the injected material. Many, but not all, of the injectable materials are radioopaque. Also, subcutaneous emphysema caused by the high-pressure injection may be appreciated. Immediate surgical consultation is required and the emergency physician should recognize this injury as potentially limb-threatening and the definitive treatment to maximize recovery and functional outcome is surgical decom-pression and debridement.

Further reading

1 Vasilevski D, Noorbergen M, Depierreux M, Lafontaine M. High-pressure injection injuries to the hand. *Am J Emerg Med* 2000; **18**(7):820–4.
2 Gutowski KA, Chu J, Choi M, Friedman DW. High-pressure hand injection injuries caused by dry cleaning solvents: case reports, review of the literature, and treatment guidelines. *Plast Reconstr Surg* 2003;**111**(1):174–7.
3 Barr ST, Wittenborn W, Nguyen D, Beatty E. High-pressure cement injection injury of the hand: a case report. *J Hand Surg* 2002;**27**(2):347–9.

Case 62 | Chest pain in a middle-aged male patient with ST segment elevation

Answer: C

Diagnosis: ST segment elevation secondary to benign early repolarization

Discussion: The 12-lead electrocardiogram (ECG) in this case demonstrates a normal sinus rhythm with ST segment elevation in the precordial leads. The elevated ST segment is concave with obvious elevation of the J point. These features are suggestive of benign early repolarization (BER).

The syndrome of BER is felt to be a normal variant, not indicative of underlying cardiac disease or increased cardio-vascular risk. BER has been reported in men and women of all age and ethnic groups; for unknown reasons, BER is seen more often in young individuals, men, and African-American persons. The mean age of patients with BER was approxi-mately 40 years with the majority of individuals being less than 50 years of age.

The ECG definition of BER includes the following character-istics: [1] ST segment elevation; [2] upward concavity of the initial portion of the ST segment; [3] notching or slurring of the terminal QRS complex; [4] symmetric, concordant T waves of large amplitude; [5] widespread or diffuse distribution of ST

segment elevation on the ECG; and [6] relative temporal sta-bility. The ST segment elevation begins at the J point with the degree of J point elevation usually less than 3.5 mm. This ST segment elevation morphologically appears as if the ST seg-ment has been evenly lifted upwards from the isoelectric base-line at the J point. This elevation results in a preservation of the normal concavity of the initial, up-sloping portion of the ST-segment–T-wave complex (a very important electrocardio-graphic feature used to distinguish BER-related ST segment elevation from STE associated with ST-elevation myocardial infarction or STEMI).

With ST segment elevation, a concave morphology of the elevated segment is more often associated with a non-STEMI cause of the ECG abnormality while a non-concave (obliquely straight or convex) shape is seen in STEMI patients. This technique uses the morphology of the initial portion of the ST-segment/T-wave, defined as beginning at the J point and ending at the apex of the T-wave (Figures 62.1C and 62.1D). Patients with non-infarctional ST segment elevation (i.e., with early repolarization, Figure 62.1C) tend to have a concave morphology of the waveform. Conversely, patients with

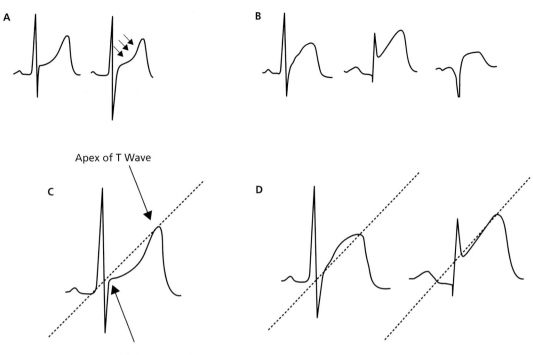

Figure 62.1 **A** ST segment elevation in benign early repolarization. Note the concave nature of the elevated ST segment (arrows). **B** ST segment elevation in STEMI. Note the convex or obliquely straight morphology of the elevated ST segment. **C** Determination of the morphology of the elevated ST segment in benign early repolarization. The J point and apex of the T wave are located; a line is drawn through these two points. If the ST segment is below the line, then a non-STEMI cause of ST segment elevation is likely. **D** Determination of the morphology of the elevated ST segment in STEMI. A line is drawn through the J point and the apex of the T wave; if the ST segment is above or superimposed on the ST segment, then STEMI is a likely explanation of the elevated ST segment.

ST segment elevation due to STEMI have either obliquely flat or convex waveforms (grouped together as non-concave, Figure 62.1D). The use of this ST segment elevation waveform analysis in ED chest pain patients is a very specific clinical tool – meaning that it should be used to rule in patients with STEMI. It must be stressed that this technique is not sensitive; it should not be used as a justification alone for ruling out a STEMI. This morphologic observation should only be used as a guideline. As with most guidelines, it is not perfect. Atypical patterns of STEMI can present with a concave pattern while non-infarction causes of ST segment elevation can manifest a non-concave morphology of the elevated segment.

Further reading

1 Brady WJ. Benign early repolarization: electrocardiographic manifestations and differentiation from other ST segment elevation syndromes. *Am J Emerg Med* 1998;**16**:592–7.
2 Brady WJ, Syverud SA, Beagle C, *et al*. Electrocardiographic ST segment elevation: the diagnosis of AMI by morphologic analysis of the ST segment. *Acad Emerg Med* 2001;**8**:961–7.

Case 63 | **Deformed globe following trauma**

Answer: D
Diagnosis: Globe rupture
Discussion: A history of blunt trauma to the orbital region with an exam showing total hyphema (also called eight-ball or blackball hyphema), severe subconjunctival hemorrhage, and limited extraocular muscle mobility suggests serious intraocular injury. When the mechanism of injury or exam findings are concerning for globe rupture, appropriate treatment should be initiated and continued until the diagnosis is reliably excluded. Globe rupture represents an ophthalmologic emergency and management is surgical in practically all cases.

Any injury that violates the integrity of ocular structures by perforation, penetration, and/or intraocular foreign body constitutes an open-globe injury. Findings suggestive of globe rupture or an open-globe injury include a peaked or irregular pupil, scleral buckling, intraocular contents found outside of globe, full thickness scleral or corneal lacerations, prolapse or distortion of the iris, traumatic cataract, traumatic lens subluxation or dislocation, either a shallow or deep anterior chamber (compared to the other side), vitreous hemorrhage, and enophthalmos or exophthalmos (with associated retro-bulbar hemorrhage). The appearance of an ooze of fluorescent fluid, under cobalt-blue light, from the corneal surface after fluorescein staining represents an aqueous humor leak from a full thickness injury (positive Siedel test).

Management of the patient with suspected globe rupture should begin with protection of the injured eye with a rigid shield. It is critical to avoid putting any pressure on or around the globe to minimize the chance of extrusion of intraocular contents. Therefore soft patches, as well as measurements of intraocular pressure, are contraindicated when considering a globe rupture. Once the diagnosis is entertained, no further palpation or manipulation of the affected eye should be undertaken until the patient is examined by ophthalmology. Prophylactic antibiotics should be started, ideally within 6 hours of the injury, to prevent the complication of endophthalmitis. Antibiotic selection may vary, but coverage for gram-positive organisms, skin flora, pseudomonas, and anaerobic organisms should be considered. Intravenous cefazolin and a fluoroquinolone have good antimicrobial coverage and intraocular penetration, and are considered reasonable initial treatment selections. Tetanus updates, analgesia, and anti-emetics should be given to avoid valsalva maneuvers with

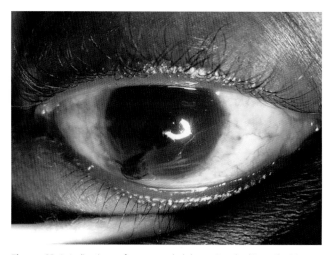

Figure 63.1 Indications of a ruptured globe: a "peaked" pupil without an afferent pupillary defect, mild conjunctival chemosis, a corneal laceration with prolapsed iris tissue, and a shallow anterior chamber.

associated increased intraocular pressure. Computerized tomography (CT) scanning of the orbits is the most sensitive and accessible imaging study to diagnose rupture, detect foreign bodies, and visualize the relevant anatomy.

Further reading

1 Aldave AJ, Gertner GS, Davis GH, *et al.* Bungee cord-associated ocular trauma. *Ophthalmology* 2001;**108**(4):788–92.
2 Monolopolous J. Emergency primary eye care. Tips for diagnosis and acute management. *Aust Fam Phys* 2002;**31**(3):233–7.

Case 64 | **Adult male with atraumatic lower back pain and leg weakness**

Answer: D

Diagnosis: Cauda equina syndrome

Discussion: Cauda equina syndrome (CES) is a neurologic disorder that is caused by compression of the spinal nerve roots comprising the cauda equina, the terminus of the spinal cord. CES presents classically with lower extremity weakness, perineal numbness, and bladder and/or bowel dysfunction. The usual etiology is lumbar disc herniation; other causes include metastasis to the spine, hematoma, abscess, fracture with fragment compression, and transverse myelitis. The typical patient is an adult male in the fourth and fifth decades with disc herniation and a history of recent lower back discomfort; less commonly, patients will present with simultaneous new onset back pain and CES. CES is an uncommon presentation with one in 2500 lower back pain patients exhibiting the syndrome.

The history reveals lower back pain associated with lower extremity weakness, perineal numbness, and bladder and/or

bowel dysfunction. The physical examination demonstrates combined motor and sensory deficits. Neurologic deficits include bilateral leg weakness, positive straight leg raise, decreased deep tendon reflexes, saddle anesthesia, and bladder retention or incontinence. Three bedside maneuvers will assist the clinician in the consideration of CES, including a rectal examination, post-void residual (PVR), and straight leg raise. The rectal examination, assessing perineal sensation and anal sphincter tone, is the first important step. Then, a PVR should be measured; values greater than 100 mL of urine should prompt concern. Urinary retention is both sensitive and specific for the diagnosis. Lastly, a straight leg raise should be attempted to further evaluate for suspected radicular symptoms.

The suspicion for the diagnosis is raised by an awareness of the syndrome coupled with clinical suspicion for CES. Confirmatory evidence is supplied by advanced radiographic imaging. Initially, a plain view radiograph is performed to rule

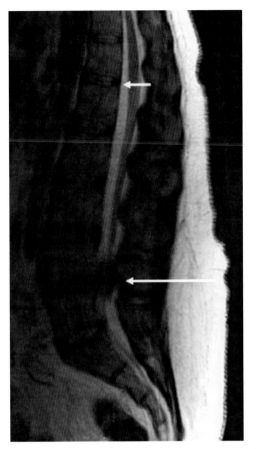

Figure 64.1 The MRI of the clinical case. There is herniation of the L4 disc with compression (large arrow) of the spinal nerve roots (cauda equina). The normal disc position at the T12 level is shown with the small arrow.

out lumbar fracture and this film will likely be normal or non-specifically abnormal in this presentation. Additional appropriate imaging includes magnetic resonance imaging (MRI) scanning. Ideally, all patients with suspected CES should undergo MRI of the spine for confirmation and localization of the lesion. If MRI is not available, then CT-myelography is an alternative imaging tool.

In the emergency department, treatment should include intravenous steroids and surgical consultation. Steroid therapy is recommended early in the course of evaluation; dexamethasone at a dose of 6–8 mg is a reasonable choice. Surgical consultation, either from a neurosurgeon or orthopedic spine surgeon, should also be performed. The urgency with which the surgeon decides on operative management is clearly not a decision made by the emergency clinician. Controversy exists within the surgical community regarding the urgency of operation. Most authors agree that early surgical intervention is the best approach with "early" defined as occurring within the first 48 hours after diagnosis. Other surgeons feel that urgent surgery at the time of diagnosis is the most appropriate. It is widely believed that patients who have earlier operations have decreased neurologic disability. Unfortunately, many patients are left with permanent deficits. In general, the patient is likely to be discharged from the hospital with the same neurologic status present as was noted at the time of surgery.

Further reading

1 Shapiro S. Medical realities of cauda equina syndrome secondary to lumbar disc herniation. *Spine* 2000;**25**:348–51.
2 Hussain SA, Gullan RW, Chitnavis BP. Cauda equina syndrome: outcome and implications for management. *Br J Neurosurg* 2003; **17**:164–7.

Case 65 | **Fever and rash in a child**

Answer: D
Diagnosis: Kawasaki disease
Discussion: Kawasaki disease (KD) is a systemic vasculitis occurring most commonly in the pediatric population. Data from the United States reveal a male preponderance (1.5–1.7:1), 76% of cases occurring before age 5, and a median age of diagnosis and hospitalization at age 2 years. It is currently the most common cause of acquired heart disease in children in the United States. The most feared complication of this disease is coronary artery aneurysms or ectasia which develop in about 15–25% of untreated children. KD's exact etiology remains unknown.

The challenge in the diagnosis of KD is that it is a clinical diagnosis with no specific laboratory testing available. To meet the classic diagnosis of KD, a patient must have fever for 5 days or more and at least four of the following five clinical symptoms: polymorphous rash (often erythematous and maculopapular); inflammatory changes of the lips and mouth (strawberry tongue, red lips that are dry and cracked; diffuse erythema of the oral or pharyngeal mucosa that is generally without exudates); bilateral conjunctivits that is nonexudative; changes in the extremities including edema, erythema of the palms and soles, and (2–3 weeks into the course) peeling of the fingers and toes. Some of these symptoms may be transient and require a careful history. Children with prolonged fever and less than four of the above symptoms may still have coronary artery abnormalities and are considered "atypical" KD. Children <1 year of age often have an atypical presentation and are also at greater risk for developing cardiac sequelae.

Besides these classic findings, there are other clinical and laboratory findings that have been reported with KD. Children invariably will have an elevated erythrocyte sedimentation rate (ESR). A urinalysis often reveals a sterile pyuria. An elevated platelet count is also common with KD. Hydrops of the gallbladder, while not specific to KD, has also been reported with ultrasound in some of these patients. When KD is clinically suspected, an echocardiogram should be performed at the time of diagnosis to look for coronary artery abnormalities.

Prompt treatment with intravenous immunoglobulin (IVIG) combined with higher, anti-inflammatory doses of aspirin in the acute phase of the illness (generally within 10 days of fever onset) decreases the risk of coronary artery abnormalities

to <5%. Once persistently afebrile, the amount of aspirin given is lowered to an anti-platelet dose. This dose of aspirin is generally maintained until follow-up echocardiograms are performed. The exact role and dosing schedule of aspirin in the treatment of these cases is still debated.

Further reading

1 Royle J, Burgner D, Curtis N. The diagnosis and management of Kawasaki disease. *J Paediatr Child Health* 2005;**41**(3):87–93.
2 Newburger JW, Fulton DR. Kawasaki disease. *Curr Opin Pediatr* 2004;**16**(5):508–14.

Case 66 | **Yellow eyes and skin**

Answer: B

Diagnosis: Jaundice secondary to hyperbilirubinemia

Discussion: The first step in the diagnosis of jaundice is determining the type of hyperbilirubinemia. Blood should be analyzed for levels of conjugated and unconjugated bilirubin, alanine aminotransferase, aspartate aminotransferase, alkaline phosphatase, and gamma-glutamyltransferase. If unconjugated bilirubin is elevated primarily, then a disorder of bilirubin metabolism should be suspected. Increased bilirubin production occurs from hemolysis, ineffective erythropoiesis, massive transfusion, or resorption of large hematomas. Decreased hepatocelluar uptake can be caused by drugs such as rifampin. Decreased conjugation is caused by Gilbert's or Crigler–Najjar syndrome and is the cause of physiologic jaundice of the newborn.

If the hyperbilirubinemia is predominantly conjugated, etiology is likely to be secondary to liver disease, cholestasis, extrinsic bile duct compression, Dubin–Johnson, or Rotor's syndrome. Alanine aminotransferease and aspartate aminotransferase elevation suggests intrinsic liver disease or a cholestatic process. Normal to mildly elevated transaminases, with an elevated alkaline phosphate and gamma-glutamyltransferase suggests extrinsic bile duct compression. Etiologies of intrinsic liver disease include hepatitis, cirrhosis, hepatotoxins, metabolic disorders of the liver such as Wilson's disease,

HELLP syndrome, and infiltrative diseases like amyloidosis and metastatic carcinoma. Cholestatic diseases include graft versus host disease, primary biliary cirrhosis and drugs such as erythromycin and chlorpromazine.

Extrinsic obstruction of the bile ducts can be caused by cholelithiasis and cholecystitis, primary sclerosing cholangitis, postsurgical strictures, neoplasms of the pancreatic head and biliary tract, and pancreatitis. The classic diagnosis associated with painless jaundice is pancreatic carcinoma. Courvoisier's sign is painless enlargement of the gallbladder that represents extrinsic compression of the biliary tree, however it is present in less than a third of patients with biliary obstruction. Initial imaging of the right upper quadrant can be done with either computerized tomography or ultrasound. Further workup should be directed by the outcome of initial lab values and abdominal imaging. Scleral icterus is more sensitive than jaundice for the detection of hyperbilirubinemia because of the high concentration of elastin in the sclera which has a high affinity for bilirubin. Vitamin A toxicity does not cause scleral icterus.

Further reading

1 Akobeng A. Neonatal jaundice. *Clin Evid* 2004;(12):501–7.
2 O'Regan D, Tait P. Imaging of the jaundiced patient. *Hosp Med* 2005;**66**(1):17–22.

Case 67 | **Fishing in the stomach**

Answer: B

Diagnosis: Lead foreign body retained in the stomach

Discussion: Serious lead poisoning has been associated with either massive lead foreign body ingestions or prolonged

retention of foreign bodies in the gastrointestinal tract. There are fatalities from lead foreign bodies retained in the gastrointestinal tract. There are also reports of markedly elevated blood lead levels within 24 hours following ingestion of large lead foreign bodies or multiple lead foreign bodies. Endoscopic removal should be performed when children present with lead foreign bodies retained within the stomach to avoid these complications.

There are numerous myths and antiquated practices associated with gastrointestinal decontamination following toxin ingestion. Home use of syrup of ipecac has been abandoned and it is inappropriate to administer it in the emergency department. The use of gastric lavage is rarely indicated in the management of the poisoned patient. Studies have failed to demonstrate a clinical benefit from the use of gastric lavage in the overdose setting. Gastric lavage is certainly not indicated in this case as the fishing weight is too large to remove by lavage. Whole bowel irrigation (WBI) involves the enteral administration of an osmotically balanced polyethylene glycol–electrolyte solution in a sufficient amount and rate to physically flush ingested substances through the gastrointestinal tract. It has been theorized, though not definitively proven, that toxins ingested may be purged with WBI before absorption can occur. WBI is not indicated in this case as the object ingested is too large to pass the pylorus (Figure 67.1). Activated charcoal (AC) is still utilized in the emergency department for the decontamination of the gastrointestinal tract. It acts by adsorbing a wide range of toxins. It also acts by enhancing toxin elimination, if systemic absorption has already occurred, by creating a concentration gradient between the contents of the bowel and the circulation. AC also has the potential of interrupting enterohepatic circulation if the particular toxin is secreted in the bile and enters the gastrointestinal tract prior to reabsorption. Single dose AC is indicated if the clinician estimates that a clinically significant fraction of the ingested substance remains in the gastrointestinal tract, the toxin is adsorbed by

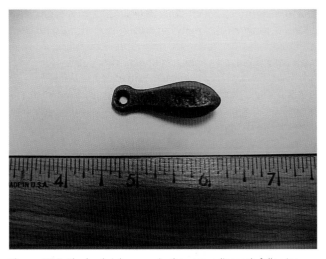

Figure 67.1 The lead sinker seen in the case radiograph following endoscopic recovery.

charcoal, and further absorption may result in clinical deterioration. AC is most effective within the first 60 minutes after oral overdose and decreases in effectiveness over time. AC is contraindicated in any patient with a compromised airway, after an ingestion of a corrosive substance (acid or alkali), and in cases where the toxin does not adsorb to AC. AC is not indicated in this case as lead is not adsorbed by AC.

Further reading

1 Heard K. Gastrointestinal decontamination. *Med Clin North Am* 2005;**89**(6):1067–78.
2 McKinney PE. Acute elevation of blood lead levels within hours of ingestion of large quantities of lead shot. *J Toxicol Clin Toxicol* 2000;**38**(4):435–40.

Case 68 | **Agitation in a botanist**

Answer: A

Diagnosis: Anticholinergic syndrome by Jimson weed (*Datura stramonium*)

Discussion: The physical exam is consistent with anticholinergic poisoning. In this particular case, the patient ingested a tea brewed from Jimson weed (*Datura stramonium*) seeds. Each seed of Jimson weed contains atropine and has been used since colonial times as both an herbal medicine and a drug of abuse. A key feature that differentiates this clinical syndrome from sympathomimetic toxicity would be the absence of sweating, presence of urinary retention, and loss of bowel sounds. Anticholinergic drugs or plants competitively bind to and block the muscarinic receptors. Anticholinergic agent ingestion can cause confusion,

agitation, hallucinations, anhydrosis, mydriasis, cycloplegia, tachycardia, fever, hypertension, urinary retention, and ileus. Anticholinergic toxicity is described by the phrase, *"Mad as a hatter, red as a beet, dry as a bone, blind as a bat, and hot as a hare."*

The differential diagnosis for the anticholinergic syndrome is broad and includes multiple plants (i.e. deadly nightshade), mushrooms, and drugs (i.e. diphenhydramine, phenothiazines). The death cap mushroom (*Amanita phalloides*) is not anticholinergic and contains a potent hepatotoxin. Patients who ingest these mushrooms do not present with an anticholinergic syndrome; instead, they present with delayed vomiting, dehydration, and potentially progress to fulminant liver failure.

The majority of anticholinergic poisonings typically have good outcomes with simply supportive care along with benzodiazepines for agitation. In the extreme cases of poisoning with anticholinergic agents, patients can develop rhabdomyolysis, marked hyperthermia, and extreme agitation.

Anticholinergic agents may also interfere with other receptors than just muscarinic receptors. For example, cyclic antidepressants inhibit cardiac sodium channels causing prolongation of the QRS complex, phenothiazines inhibit cardiac potassium efflux channels causing QT prolongation, and diphenhydramine inhibits histamine receptors resulting in seizures.

Further reading

1 Vanderhoff BT, Mosser KH. Jimson weed toxicity: management of anticholinergic plant ingestion. *Am Fam Physician* 1992;**46**(2): 526–30.
2 Dyer S. Plant exposures: wilderness medicine. *Emerg Med Clin North Am* 2004;**22**(2):299–313.

Case 69 | **Skin target lesion**

Answer: B

Diagnosis: Erythema migrans from Lyme disease

Discussion: This is an example of the target lesion erythema migrans (EM), associated with Lyme disease (LD). LD is the most common vector born disease in the US. It is caused by *Borrelia burgdorferi*, a spirochete, transmitted by the *Ixodes* species deer tick. LD occurs in areas where there is an abundance of deer ticks and the percentage of infected ticks is high. The highest incidence of LD in the US is found in northeastern, north-central, and western states. Connecticut followed by Rhode Island, New York, New Jersey, Delaware, Pennsylvania, Maryland, Massachusetts, and Wisconsin account for the vast majority of cases reported.

The transmission risk is directly related to the duration of feed. Nymphs (responsible for 85% of transmission) require 36–48 hours of a blood meal for transmission, whereas adults require 48–72 hours. This would require that the tick be attached and engorged if found on the skin. Overall, the risk for LD after a tick bite in endemic areas has been shown to be only approximately 3%. These ticks not only carry LD, but also can carry *Babesia microti* and *Ehrlichia equi.*

The inoculation of *B. burgdorferi* into the skin leads to a local inflammatory reaction leading to the characteristic target lesion, EM. This is the only pathognomonic feature of LD, and it is sufficient to diagnose the disease. It typically appears as a flat erythematous lesion with reinforced borders, which expands with a constant diameter over a period of days. It can appear solid, ring shaped with central clearing or as a bull's eye. It appears at the site of attachment of the tick while the spirochetes are confined to the skin. Occasionally vesicles and/or necrotic areas may occur at the center of the lesion leading to pain in the usually asymptomatic lesion. The appearance of EM usually signifies the *"Early localized"* phase of disease, within the first 3–30 days after the tick bite, which may also be accompanied by regional lymphadenopathy and constitutional flu-like symptoms. EM will resolve on its own, even without treatment, over several weeks and the vast majority go unnoticed. In the emergency department, it is important to differentiate EM from other conditions such as cellulitis, nummular eczema, granuloma annulare, ring worm, or an insect bite.

If the host's immune system does not contain the spirochete locally, hematogenous spread leads to *"Early disseminated"* disease. This stage may also present with EM, which may be single or multiple. Additional symptoms include constitutional symptoms, meningitis, carditis, cranial neuritis, and radiculoneuritis. This phase is seen 3–12 weeks after the tick bite. Finally, *"Late disease"* is seen greater than 2 months after the tick bite and is usually characterized as arthritis and/or central nervous system involvement. Lyme arthritis is the most common manifestation of LD that presents to the emergency department. It is usually mono- or oligoarticular and commonly presents with intermittent swelling of the knee, ankle and/or elbow joints.

The treatment of choice for patients with early localized disease above 8 years of age is doxycycline. Children 8 years of age or younger should be treated with amoxicillin (50 mg/ kg/day) to avoid the potential side effect of staining the enamel of pre-erupted teeth. For patients with LD with any associated central nervous system or cardiac involvement, intravenous therapy with ceftriaxone is recommended.

Prevention is as important as treatment in controlling this disease. A daily skin check in endemic areas is one of the best methods of prevention of spread of the disease. Immediate tick removal should be performed with care.

Further reading

1 DePietropaolo DL, Powers JH, Gil JM, Foy AJ. Diagnosis of lyme disease. *Am Fam Physician* 2005;**72**(2):297–304.
2 Edlow JA. Lyme disease and related tick-borne illnesses. *Ann Emerg Med* 1999;**33**(6):680–93.
3 Bachman DT, Srivastava G. Emergency department presentations of Lyme disease in children. *Pediatr Emerg Care* 1998;**14**(5): 356–61.

Case 70 | **Adult male with a sudden, severe headache**

Answer: E

Diagnosis: Subarachnoid hemorrhage

Discussion: A non-traumatic subarachnoid hemorrhage (SAH) most commonly results from a ruptured aneurysm (80% of the time) within the subarachnoid space and leads to the death or disability of 18,000 people in North America annually. Aneurysms are acquired lesions from vascular stresses at bifurcations or bends of arteries; rupture is more likely in people with hypertension, those who smoke or drink alcohol, and those with multiple or enlarging aneurysms. The median age for a SAH is 50 years of age and there is a 2.1 times increased incidence in African-Americans than in whites and a slightly higher incidence in women than in men.

The typical presentation of a SAH is the acute onset of a severe "thunderclap" headache that is classically described as "the worst headache of my life." As many as 30–50% of patients will report sentinel headaches over the proceeding weeks to months that result from the slow leakage of blood. Signs of meningeal irritation are seen in over 75% of patients although it may take several hours for these symptoms to manifest. One-half of patients will experience loss of consciousness at the onset of the bleed and between one-tenth and one-quarter will experience a seizure within an hour of onset. Nausea, vomiting and photophobia are also common presenting symptoms. About 50% of patients will have increased blood pressure at the time of presentation from the Cushing response. The physical exam may be normal, but approximately one-quarter will have non-focal neurological abnormalities. Papilledema or subhyloid retinal hemorrhages may be present on fundoscopic exam.

A non-contrast head computerized tomography (CT) is indicated as the diagnostic test of choice in all patients with suspected SAH and is most sensitive at 24 hours after the onset but will be falsely negative in as many as 10–15% of patients. A lumbar puncture should be considered when there is a high clinical suspicion but a negative head CT; lumbar puncture is positive when there is a consistently elevated number of red blood cells in two consecutive tubes of cerebrospinal fluid (CSF) or if xanthochromia, the resulting CSF color change from red blood cell degradation, is present. A lumbar puncture may be falsely negative less than 2 hours after the onset of bleeding and is most sensitive 12 hours after the bleed. Once the diagnosis is made, neurosurgical consultation with cerebral angiography should be obtained to assess the status of the bleeding. Patients should be considered for non-sedating seizure prophylaxis and calcium channel blockers that reduce the incidence of cerebral vasospasm. A goal mean blood pressure of less than 130 mmHg should be obtained with antihypertensive agents. If herniation is suspected, mannitol or furosemide can be used to reduce intracranial pressure. The prognosis of patients with SAH is poor; between 10 and 15% will die before reaching the hospital, 40% will die within a week, and over half will die within 6 months.

Further reading

1 Edlow JA. Diagnosis of subarachnoid hemorrhage. *Neurocrit Care* 2005;**2**(2):99–109.
2 Le Roux PD, Winn HR. Management of the ruptured aneurysm. *Neurosurg Clin North Am* 1998;**9**(3):525–40.
3 Liebenberg WA, Worth R, Firth GB. Aneurysmal subarachnoid haemorrhage: guidance in making the correct diagnosis. *Postgrad Med J* 2005;**81**(957):470–3.

Case 71 | **Get them undressed!**

Answer: C

Diagnosis: Meningococcemia

Discussion: *Neisseria meningitidis* is an encapsulated gram negative diploccus that is a strict human pathogen. Meningococci can cause a clinical presentation ranging from mild illness to fulminant disease. The duration of symptoms ranges from less than 12 hours to greater than 14 days. Petechiae or purpura with fever are the classical findings of meningococcemia. Other findings include headache, neck stiffness, hyperthermia, hypothermia, hypotension, arthritis, seizures, irritability, lethargy, emesis, diarrhea, cough, and rhinorrhea.

The skin should be carefully examined for the presence of lesions, which may be the only clue of meningococcemia. Petechiae are present in 50–60% of cases, but macular and maculopapular nodules are also common. Septic shock with petechiae or purpura indicates endotoxin release and/or disseminated intravascular coagulation. Other causes of petechiae include thrombotic thrombocytopenic purpura, idiopathic thrombocytopenic purpura, blunt trauma, cirrhosis, nutritional deficiencies, chemotherapy, or thrombocytopenia of other origin.

Initial therapy includes placing the patient in isolation, administering immediate antibiotics, and drawing appropriate cultures. Transmission occurs via infected secretions necessitating droplet isolation precautions. Because meningococcus can have such a rapidly progressive course, antibiotics should be administered as soon as possible. Our patient shows evidence of septic shock and thus should receive antibiotics without standard delays, including head computerized tomography (CT) and lumbar puncture. Cultures, including blood and cerebrospinal fluid should be drawn as soon as possible to help isolate the pathogenic organism.

Further reading

1 Hazelzet JA. Diagnosing meningococcemia as a cause of sepsis. *Pediatr Crit Care Med* 2005;**6**(3):S50–4.
2 Kirsch EA, Barton RP, Kitchen L, Giroir BP. Pathophysiology, treatment and outcome of meningococcemia: a review and recent experience. *Pediatr Infect Dis J* 1996;**15**(11):967–78.
3 Holstege CP. Petechiae and purpura associated with meningococcemia. *Ann Emerg Med* 2005;**45**(5):560.

Case 72 | **Chest pain and subtle ST segment elevation**

Answer: B
Diagnosis: Subtle STEMI with reciprocal change
Discussion: The patient's 12-lead electrocardiogram (ECG) demonstrates subtle ST segment elevation in the inferior leads. The presence of ST segment depression in leads I and aVl, known as reciprocal ST segment depression or reciprocal change, confirms that the subtle ST segment elevation in the inferior leads results from ST-elevation myocardial infarction (STEMI).

Reciprocal ST segment depression, also known as reciprocal change, is defined as STD in leads separate and distinct from leads reflecting ST segment elevation. The cause of reciprocal change remains unknown but may involve: (1) displacement of the injury current vector away from the infarcting myocardium; (2) co-existing distant ischemia; and/or (3) a manifestation of infarct extension. Regardless of its cause, reciprocal change in the setting of transmural acute myocardial infarction (AMI) identifies a patient with increased chance of poor outcome and, therefore, an individual who may benefit from a more aggressive approach in the emergency department. Furthermore, its presence on the ECG supports the diagnosis of AMI with very high sensitivity and positive predictive values greater than 90%. Patients with inferior wall AMI manifest reciprocal change in approximately 75% of cases while anterior wall myocardial infarcts demonstrate such STD much less often – usually in one-third of patients.

In a large prehospital chest pain population undergoing 12-lead ECG analysis, Otto and Aufderheide reported that reciprocal ST segment depressions supported the diagnosis of AMI with both a high specificity and a high positive predictive value – both greater than 90%. In an emergency department based chest pain population, it was noted that reciprocal ST segment depression was very useful in the ECG diagnosis of STEMI with both a specificity and a positive predictive value of 93%. The presence of reciprocal changes has inadequate sensitivity to exclude STEMI, but its presence should alert the clinician of STEMI when analyzing ECGs with borderline or atypical ST segment elevations. Inferior AMI patients with precordial ST segment depression (i.e. reciprocal changes indicating extension to posterior wall) or elevation in right ventricular leads (i.e. extension to right anterior ventricular wall) have a worse prognosis and presumably benefit more from fibrinolytic agents than patients with isolated inferior ST segment elevation.

Further reading

1 Otto LA, Aufderheide TP. Evaluation of ST segment elevation criteria for the prehospital electrocardiographic diagnosis of acute myocardial infarction. *Ann Emerg Med* 1994;**23**:17–24.
2 Brady WJ, Perron AD, Syverud SA, *et al.* Reciprocal ST-segment depression: impact on the electrocardiographic diagnosis of ST-segment elevation acute myocardial infarction. *Am J Emerg Med* 2002;**20**:35–8.

Case 73 | **Fluid in my eye**

Answer: E
Diagnosis: Traumatic hyphema
Discussion: A traumatic hyphema is defined as blood in the anterior chamber of the eye usually the result of blunt globe trauma. The blood may be suspended in the aqueous

(as shown in figure on page 47), layered in the anterior chamber, or filling the entire anterior chamber. It is important to determine the mechanism of injury causing the hyphema. Complete ocular examination is important to rule out a ruptured globe. A dilated fundus examination or ultrasound should be performed to rule out posterior segment injury. A computerized tomography (CT) scan of the brain and orbits should be considered when globe rupture or intraocular foreign body is suspected.

The intraocular pressure should be measured in all patients with a hyphema provided globe rupture has been ruled out. Intraocular pressure elevation greater than 25 mmHg occurs in 25% of patients with a hyphema. The pressure elevation is due to trabecular meshwork obstruction by red blood cells or damage to the normal aqueous outflow channels. Intraocular pressure can be easily measured in the emergency department using various instruments, such as a Tono-Pen. Patients of Mediterranean or African descent patients should be screened for sickle cell trait or disease.

Treatment for hyphemas is mainly supportive unless the intraocular pressure is uncontrolled. Patients should be confined to bedrest or limited activity. Elevate the head 30 degrees. A metal shield should be placed over the injured eye at all times. Atropine 1% ophthalmic drops should be instilled twice a day to relieve ciliary spasms and enhance patient comfort. Prednisolone acetate 1% ophthalmic suspension instilled four times a day will help suppress inflammation in the injured eye. Patients should avoid aspirin containing products.

Patients with elevated intraocular pressure can usually be managed with topical antiglaucoma therapy. Treatment is aimed at reducing aqueous production. A topical beta blocker (timolol or levobunolol 0.5%) twice a day may be combined with an alpha agonist (brimonidine 0.2%) three times a day and a topical carbonic anhydrase inhibitor (dorzolamide 2%) three times a day. If unsuccessful, oral acetazolamide 500 mg twice a day may be added. However, carbonic anhydrase inhibitors should be avoided in patients with sickle cell disease or trait since these medications may reduce the anterior chamber pH and induce sickling. Despite medical therapy, approximately 5% of patients with a hyphema will require surgical intervention to control their intraocular pressure. Ophthalmology consultation should be obtained for all patients with hyphema since these patients will require long-term monitoring for development of glaucoma.

Further reading
1 Walton W, Von Hagen S, Grigorian R, Zarbin M. Management of traumatic hyphema. *Surv Ophthalmol* 2002;**47**(4):297–334.
2 Sankar PS, Chen TC, Grosskreutz CL, Pasquale LR. Traumatic hyphema. *Int Ophthalmol Clin* 2002;**42**(3):57–68.

Case 74 | Coma following head trauma

Answer: D
Diagnosis: Epidural hematoma
Discussion: An epidural hematoma (EDH) is the accumulation of blood in the space between the dura and the inner surface of the skull that results from trauma in 85–90% of cases. The temperoparietal region is the area most commonly fractured (66–80% of the time) which results in damage to the underlying middle meningeal artery or one of its dural branches. The extravasation of blood is limited by the suture lines due to the attachment of the dura to the skull at these points. EDHs are most common in people less than 20 years old (60% of cases); EDHs are rare in children less than 2 years of age because the skull is soft and less likely to fracture and rare in adults older than 50 where the dura is more tightly adherent to the skull.

The classic "lucid interval" between the initial loss of consciousness at the time of injury and a delayed decline of level of consciousness is seen in less than a third of cases. Posterior fossa EDHs are associated with a delayed but extremely rapid deterioration of mental status that can quickly progress to coma or death in only a matter of minutes. The most common presenting signs and symptoms are severe headache, nausea, seizure, and occasionally focal neurological deficits. On examination, the Cushing response from increased intracranial pressure might result in hypertension and bradycardia. Lacerations, contusions, or bony step-offs indicative of underlying skull fracture are common but not always present. Dilated, sluggish, or fixed pupils bilaterally or ipsilaterally to the side of injury are concerning for increased intracranial pressure and impending herniation.

An emergent head computed tomography (CT) without contrast is indicated in all patients with suspicion for an EDH. Acute EDHs may appear as a lens-shaped hypodensity between the skull and brain parenchyma – a convex, bulging outward contour. Lumbar puncture is not indicated. Once the diagnosis is made, immediate neurosurgical consultation is needed. Small EDHs can be treated conservatively, but larger or unstable EDHs require surgical evacuation. Signs of increased intracranial pressure should be managed by elevating the head of the bed to 30 degrees once the C-spine is cleared, assuring an adequate blood pressure, and administrating mannitol at a dose 0.25–1.0 g/kg intravenous. Intubated patients should be ventilated at 16–20 breaths/minute with a tidal volume of 10–12 mL/kg to maintain a carbon dioxide partial pressure of 28–32 mmHg. Prognosis is usually excellent with early intervention with mortality rates ranging from 0% in preoperatively non-comatosed patients to 20–40% in those in a coma before surgery.

Further reading

1 Ibanez J, Arikan F, Pedraza S. Reliability of clinical guidelines in the detection of patients at risk following mild head injury: results of a prospective study. *J Neurosurg* 2004;**100**(5):825–34.

2 Lee EJ, Hung YC, Wang LC. Factors influencing the functional outcome of patients with acute epidural hematomas: analysis of 200 patients undergoing surgery. *J Trauma* 1998;**45**(5):946–52.

Case 75 | **Blue hue following endoscopy**

Answer: D

Diagnosis: Methemoglobinemia

Discussion: Methemoglobinemia occurs when the iron atom within the hemoglobin molecule is oxidized from the ferrous (Fe^{2+}) to the ferric (Fe^{3+}) form. This results in impaired oxygen and carbon dioxide carrying capacity that can lead to a functional anemia and tissue hypoxia. It most commonly occurs as the result of exposure to oxidizing compounds or their metabolites (such as in this case, the patient received benzocaine during endoscopy), but can also result from genetic, dietary, or idiopathic causes. Methemoglobin (MHb) renders the blood a chocolate color, which is pathognomonic at the bedside. Non-anemic healthy patients can tolerate MHb levels up to 15% without symptoms. Levels between 20% and 30% may result in anxiety, tachycardia, changes in mental status and headache. MHb levels above 50% may cause coma, seizures, dysrhythmias, and death. However, cases of patients with levels greater than 70% have been reported with minimal symptoms.

The most important mechanism for prevention of methemoglobinemia in humans is the nicotinamide adenine dinucleotide (NADH) dependent methemoglobin reductase system (Figure 75.1). This enzyme is responsible for the removal of the majority of MHb that is produced under normal circumstances. The other enzyme, nicotinamide adenine dinucleotide phosphate (NADPH) methemoglobin reductase, is a minor pathway for the removal of MHb under normal conditions. However, when high concentrations of MHb are present, the NADH enzyme pathway becomes saturated and the NADPH enzyme system becomes dominant.

Cyanosis occurs in patients when as little as 1.5 g/dL of hemoglobin is in the MHb form, whereas 5 g/dL of deoxyhemoglobin is required to produce cyanosis. Pulse oximetry is misleading when MHb is present. Pulse oximetry only measures the relative absorbance of two wavelengths of light, thereby differentiating only oxyhemoglobin from deoxyhemoglobin. At high levels of MHb, the pulse oximeter reads a saturation of approximately 85%, which corresponds to equal absorbance of both wavelengths. The partial pressure of oxygen on the arterial blood gas reflects plasma oxygen content and does not correspond to the oxygen carrying capacity of hemoglobin. Therefore, in patients with MHb, their partial pressure of oxygen remains within the normal reference range. Co-oximetry should be requested to measure the

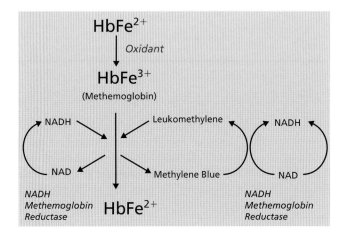

Figure 75.1 The enzymatic pathways to reduce methemoglobin.

MHb level. Co-oximetry can measure the relative absorbance of four different wavelengths of light and can thereby differentiate MHb from carboxyhemoglobin, oxyhemoglobin, and deoxyhemoglobin.

Once the diagnosis has been made, treatment is supportive for patients with minimal signs or symptoms. For symptomatic patients, methylene blue is the treatment of choice. Methylene blue is dosed at 1–2 mg/kg of a 1% solution, infused intravenously over 3–5 minutes. This dose can be repeated at 30 minutes if there is no improvement in symptoms. Methylene blue is an effective electron donor for NADPH methemoglobin reductase enzyme, thereby speeding the conversion of iron from the ferric (Fe^{3+}) to the ferrous (Fe^{2+}). Methylene blue when infused can cause burning at the site of injection. The intravenous line should be flushed promptly after injection. Methylene blue may also result in a false lowering of the pulse oximetry saturation readings.

Further reading

1 Ash-Bernal R, Wise R, Wright SM. Acquired methemoglobinemia: a retrospective series of 138 cases at 2 teaching hospitals. *Medicine (Baltimore)* 2004;**83**(5):265–73.

2 Henretig FM, Gribetz B, Kearney T, Lacouture P, Lovejoy FH. Interpretation of color change in blood with varying degree of methemoglobinemia. *J Toxicol Clin Toxicol* 1988;**26**:293–301.

3 Wright RO, Lewander WJ, Woolf AD. Methemoglobinemia: etiology, pharmacology, and clinical management. *Ann Emerg Med* 1999; **34**(5):646–56.

Case 76 | Shoulder pain following direct blow

Answer: D

Diagnosis: Type II acromioclavicular (AC) separation

Discussion: The AC joint stabilizes the scapula and gleno-humeral joint in relation to the thorax. It forms the only direct, bony connection between the arm and the thorax and axial skeleton. The AC joint is stabilized by several structures: the AC joint capsule and ligaments; the coracoacromial (CA) ligament; the coracoclavicular (CC) ligament, consisting of the conoid and trapezoid portions. AC separation is better thought of as a joint sprain and is the result of a direct blow to the adducted arm or an indirect result of a fall on the outstretched hand (FOOSH) injury. The severity of injury to the AC joint depends upon the number of these structures damaged. AC separations are classified by the Rockwood classification into Types I to VI. A Type I AC separation (partial or complete disruption of the AC ligament) reveals tenderness to palpation over the AC joint on physical examination but the radiographs are normal. X-rays of a Type II AC separation (complete disruption of the AC ligament and partial disruption of the CC ligaments) reveals displacement of the distal clavicle in relation to the acromion. This separation can range from a few percent to 100 percent. When the displacement is greater than 100% the injury is a Type III AC separation, with complete disruption of the AC and CC joints. Types IV–VI are uncommon and the lateral clavicle is widely displaced from the acromium due to disruption of either the periosteum of the clavicle or the deltoid or trapezius muscles.

Management of AC separations is usually symptomatic and non-operative. All orthopedic injuries require careful evaluation to rule out accompanying injuries. Type I separations are treated with analgesia, ice, a sling for comfort, and a brief period of immobilization, followed by progressive strengthening and range-of-motion (ROM) exercises. Type II AC separations in the past were further evaluated with "weighted X-rays," where the patient held a 10 lb weight in the hand on the injured side to maximize the degree of displacement between the clavicle and the acromium and rule out occult Type III separations. Generally, these studies have been abandoned because they can be extremely painful and do not alter

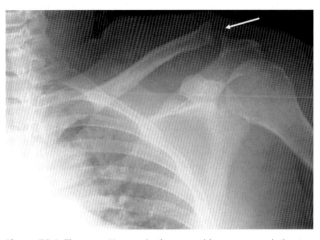

Figure 76.1 The same X-ray as in the case with an arrow pointing to the Type II AC separation (approximately 50% separation).

management. The general consensus is that Type II injuries should be managed the same as Type I. Indications for orthopedic consultation and/or operative repair include Types III–VI AC separations, significant tenting of the skin, and open AC separations. The latter of these injuries are rare. There is controversy about the management of Type III AC separations, with some shoulder specialists favoring conservative management and others favoring operative repair. Types IV–VI require operative intervention. Figure eight immobilization is not indicated in the management of AC separations. In the past, figure eight bandages were routinely used in the management of clavicle fractures, but their use has been abandoned because they are difficult for the patient to wear and the fractures frequently become displaced again as soon as the figure eight immobilizer is discontinued.

Further reading

1 Bossart PJ, Joyce SM, Manaster BJ, Packer SM. Lack of efficacy of "weighted" radiographs in diagnosing acute acromioclavicular separation. *Ann Emerg Med* 1988;**17**(1):20–4.

2 Schlegel TF, Burks RT, Marcus RL, Dunn HK. A prospective evaluation of untreated acute grade III acromioclavicular separations. *Am J Sport Med* 2001;**29**(6):699–703.

Case 77 | An overdose of prenatal vitamins

Answer: A

Diagnosis: Iron toxicity

Discussion: Iron toxicity occurs from ingestion of iron supplements. The total elemental iron ingested is dependent upon the formulation ingested. Common formulations and their percent by weight of elemental iron are as follows: ferrous gluconate (12%), ferrous lactate (19%), ferrous sulfate (20%), ferrous chloride (28%), and ferrous fumarate

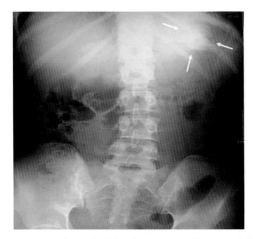

Figure 77.1 The radiograph of the chapter case with arrows delineating the radioopacity of the dissolved iron tablets in the stomach.

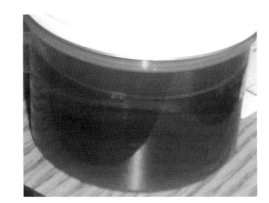

Figure 77.2 The "vin rose" urine of a patient who has iron toxicity and has been chelated with deferoxamine.

(33%). Toxic effects (gastrointestinal symptoms) generally occur at >20 mg/kg of elemental iron. Severe toxicity (shock) generally occurs at doses higher than 50 mg/kg. Five classic clinical phases have been described:

Phase 1 (0–12 hours): Gastrointestinal distress predominates initially due to iron's direct corrosive effects. Abdominal pain, diarrhea, and emesis may occur. In severe cases, hematemesis, hematochezia, large fluid losses, and shock occur.

Phase 2 (6–24 hours): A "latent" phase may be seen, where gastrointestinal symptoms subside, but end-organ toxicity continues.

Phase 3 (6–48 hours): Multisystem organ failure ensues: hypotension, depressed myocardial output, oliguria, anuria, coagulopathy, lethargy, seizures, and coma.

Phase 4 (1–4 days): Fulminant liver failure may develop.

Phase 5 (2–8 weeks): Initial gastrointestinal corrosive injury can produce pyloric and intestinal obstruction from strictures.

An iron level should be obtained and a repeat level drawn to assure iron levels are not increasing. Serum iron levels >500 μg/dL are commonly associated with systemic toxicity. Elevated white blood counts and blood glucose may be seen, but are unreliable in predicting severity of toxicity. Total iron-binding capacity (TIBC) is unreliable and should not be used to estimate free iron levels. The iron tablets may individually be visible on abdominal X-rays or may be seen as a diffuse radiopacity in the stomach (Figure 77.1). A negative X-ray does not rule out iron ingestion (i.e. children's chewable multivitamin products are not radiopaque). Iron is not the only substance known to be radiopaque. Other substances that have been reported to be radiopaque include calcium, carbon tetrachloride,

chloroform, chloral hydrate, metals (i.e. arsenic, bismuth, lead, mercury, and zinc), potassium chloride, phosphorous, phenothiazines, paradichlorobenzene mothballs, acetazolamide, sodium chloride, and spironolactone.

There is limited utility of gastrointestinal decontamination following iron overdose. Ipecac and gastric lavage are generally not recommended. Activated charcoal does not adsorb iron and should not be administered. Whole bowel irrigation may be useful, especially if tablets are visible on X-ray or levels are rising. Adequate fluid resuscitation and supportive care are the primary initial interventions. Deferoxamine is the antidote that chelates free iron. Indications include significant clinical signs of toxicity (i.e. protracted vomiting or diarrhea), metabolic acidosis, shock, serum iron levels >500 μg/dL, and/or an X-ray positive for multiple pills. Deferoxamine infusions are given intravenously at a starting rate of 15 mg/kg/hour, not to exceed 1.0 g\hour, over a total of 6 hours. The patient should then be reevaluated. Deferoxamine-induced hypotension may occur at fast rates, and adequate hydration should be assured before infusion initiation. As iron is chelated and excreted, urine will develop a characteristic rusty-red ("vin rose") appearance (Figure 77.2).

Further reading

1 Siff JE, Meldon SW, Tomassoni AJ. Usefulness of the total iron binding capacity in the evaluation and treatment of acute iron overdose. *Ann Emerg Med* 1999;**33**(1):73–6.
2 Mills KC, Curry SC. Acute iron poisoning. *Emerg Med Clin North Am* 1994;**12**(2):397–413.
3 Eldridge DL, Dobson T, Brady W, Holstege CP. Utilizing diagnostic investigations in the poisoned patient. *Med Clin North Am* 2005;**89**(6):1079–106.

Case 78 | **Fever and rash in a child**

Answer: A

Diagnosis: Neonatal herpes simplex virus (HSV) infection

Discussion: Newborns are at decidedly more risk of obtaining HSV infection from a mother who is having her first episode of genital herpes near delivery than those whose mothers are having a recurrent infection. Unfortunately, many mothers are suffering from subclinical infections and have asymptomatic viral shedding that goes undetected. As the virus has a prolonged incubation (5–21 days), a healthy-appearing neonate may be discharged from the nursery and subsequently become acutely ill. Some other risk factors for transmission from mother to neonate include the following: exposure to cervical viral shedding, low-birth-weight infants, delivery before 38 weeks gestation, use of fetal scalp electrodes, rupture of membranes >4 hours, and maternal age <21 years. Cesarean section reduces the transmission risk.

Neonatal HSV infection is classified as either localized to skin, eyes, and mouth (SEM); central nervous system (CNS) diseases; or disseminated. Disseminated disease involves multiple organ systems (including CNS, adrenal glands, skin, eyes, and mouth) but shows preference for the lungs and liver. Typically, SEM and disseminated disease presents earlier in life (10–12 days) than CNS disease presents (16–19 days). Suggestive symptoms (such as skin lesions, fever, or seizures) are not always present in disseminated and CNS disease. In fact, studies have shown that no collection of symptoms will identify all neonates with HSV infection. Many argue HSV should be particularly considered in the differential diagnosis of any acutely ill infant who is younger than 1 month of age with any of the following: seizures, unexplained acute hepatitis, typical skin lesions, septic presentation (especially with negative bacterial cultures), or the presence of HSV risk factors.

As far as diagnosis, viral culture remains the definitive modality with possible sites to culture including: skin vesicles, oropharynx, eyes, urine, blood, stool, and CSF. Polymerase chain reaction (PCR) of the CSF and blood is increasingly used due to its quick turnaround and high sensitivity and specificity. A chest radiograph and liver transaminases are also useful in disseminated disease due to HSV's affinity for the lungs and liver. Though a head computer tomography (CT) may be helpful in the setting of acute neurologic changes, in the case of HSV infection, images can appear normal early in the course.

High-dose intravenous acyclovir (60 mg/kg/day in three divided doses) is the treatment of choice for neonatal HSV infection. Mortality from CNS and disseminated HSV infection is high when untreated; therefore acyclovir should be started immediately with any *suspicion* of neonatal HSV infection.

Further reading

1 Colletti JE, Homme JL, Woodridge DP. Unsuspected neonatal killers in emergency medicine. *Emerg Med Clin North Am* 2004; **22**(4):929–960.

2 Kimberlin DW. Neonatal herpes simplex infection. *Clin Microbiol Rev* 2004;**17**(1):1–13.

3 Lewis P, Glaser CA. Encephalitis. *Pediatr Rev* 2005; **26**(10):353–63.

Case 79 | **Lamp oil ingestion**

Answer: D

Diagnosis: Hydrocarbon ingestion/aspiration

Discussion: Accidental ingestion and aspiration of hydrocarbons is a potentially fatal childhood poisoning. The likelihood of aspiration and subsequent severe lung injury correlates directly with the chemical properties of the agent ingested: surface tension, viscosity, and volatility. Low surface tension permits the hydrocarbon to spread rapidly on contact with the respiratory tract. A low viscosity leads to deeper, distal penetration of the fluid into the respiratory tract. High volatility (or greater tendency to rapidly evaporate) is thought to be damaging in two ways. First, by replacing alveolar gas with its gaseous form, the hydrocarbon can cause hypoxemia and second, by rapid systemic absorption, entry into the central nervous system, and subsequent neurological symptoms.

Clinical presentation varies in these cases. Pediatric patients who are thought to ingest a hydrocarbon should be observed closely. If no symptoms occur in 6–8 hours, they are unlikely to develop and discharge can be contemplated. Gastrointestinal effects occur from mucosal irritation and often include abdominal pain, nausea, vomiting, and diarrhea. Neurological symptoms are also common and can include dizziness, euphoria, visual disturbances, seizures, and coma. Still the respiratory symptoms are often the most prominent and concerning part of the presentation. Initial, proximal airway irritation can cause choking and coughing. With subsequent lower airway involvement, tachypnea, crackles, wheezes (bronchospasm), decreased breath sounds, retractions, grunting, and nasal flaring can develop. Fever resulting from this pulmonary insult is common. Lower respiratory symptoms and fever may develop quickly (within 30 minutes) or may be delayed for several hours. Persistent or worsening respiratory problems should be evident in 6–8 hours. Chest radiograph findings can occur as early as 30 minutes after aspiration, with nearly all manifesting within 12 hours. Initial findings can include alveolar infiltrates extending from perihilar regions to involve any segment, but predominantly involve the lower lobes. Other findings include pulmonary edema, atelectasis, and consolidation.

Persistent respiratory distress mandates admission and close observation. Treatment is largely supportive with oxygen. Bronchodilators can be used for suspected bronchospasm but conclusive proof to efficacy is lacking. Gastric lavage is strictly contraindicated as the risk of inducing vomiting and causing further aspiration is prohibitive. Activated charcoal has not been shown to bind these substances and may also lead to vomiting. Prophylactic antibiotics and steroids have not been shown to be useful or effective in the acute phase of these ingestions.

Further reading

1 Victoria MS, Nangia BS. Hydrocarbon poisoning: a review. *Pediatr Emerg Care* 1987;**3**(3):184–6.
2 Truemper E, Reyes de la Rocha S, Atkinson SD. Clinical characteristics, pathophysiology, and management of hydrocarbon ingestion: case report and review of the literature. *Pediatr Emerg Care* 1987;**3**(3):187–93.

Case 80 | Diffuse ankle pain following a fall

Answer: D
Diagnosis: Talar fracture
Discussion: The talus is the second most frequently fractured tarsal bone after the calcaneus, and fractures of this bone are generally divided into injuries of the anatomic head, neck, and body. These injuries comprise 3–5% of all foot fractures, but are likely underreported, as injuries to the talar dome frequently go unrecognized until later presentation. While injuries to the medial and lateral processes of the talus may be relatively minor, fractures through the body, neck, head, or posterior process can carry significant morbidity. The driving force in searching out these injuries is the fact that, like the scaphoid in the hand, blood supply to the talus is tenuous, and fractures that are unrecognized or inadequately treated can result in avascular necrosis (AVN) to the bone. Even when identified early and cared for properly, fractures of the talus may lead not only to AVN, but also arthritis, as well as chronic pain and non-union.

The potential for missing these injuries in the emergency department is real, as osteochondral fractures of the talar dome, posterior process fractures, and lateral process fractures all may be difficult to detect radiographically and clinically can be mistaken for ankle sprain. Talar fractures can be seen at any age, and are usually the result of motor vehicle collisions or falls from a height.

Plain radiographs of both the foot and ankle are used to diagnose talar fractures. The views obtained depend on the particular fracture. Fractures of the lateral process are especially difficult as they may be nearly invisible on the anteroposterior (AP) ankle radiograph or lateral view of the foot. Mortise views of the ankle will help to evaluate the body of the talus, as well as detect injury to the talar dome. Computerized axial tomography (CT) scan and magnetic resonance imaging (MRI) can be used to detect radiographically occult fractures of the talus as well as to determine the amount of articular surface involvement. While not required

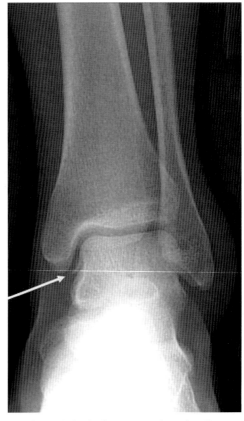

Figure 80.1 The medial talar fracture is indicated with an arrow.

in the emergency department evaluation, the clinician should have a low threshold to obtain an advanced imaging study if there is concern for occult injury or a need to determine the full extent of the fracture.

The treatment for suspected or confirmed talar fractures depends on the fracture morphology, and portion of the bone involved. Non-articular chip fractures can be treated conservatively with non-weight bearing, splinting, and sure orthopedic outpatient follow-up. Significant fractures that require orthopedic consultation in the emergency department include those through the neck (due to blood supply issues) or those with significant articular surface involvement. If there is any doubt about the diagnosis or extent of injury, advanced imaging with CT or MRI is recommended.

Further reading

1 Adelaar RS, Madrian JR. Avascular necrosis of the talus. *Orthoped Clin North Am* 2004;**35**(3):383–95.
2 Furlong J, Morrison WB, Carrino JA. Imaging of the talus. *Foot Ankle Clin* 2004;**9**(4):685–701.
3 LeBlanc KE. Ankle problems masquerading as sprains. *Prim Care* 2004;**31**(4):1055–67.

Case 81 | Emergency department drop-off

Answer: E
Diagnosis: Opioid toxicity
Discussion: The first picture on page 52 depicts a disconjugate gaze and miosis in a woman who was intoxicated with heroin. The second picture on page 52 depicts the site of where the patient injects – the axilla. Opium, a dried extract from the poppy plant *Papaver somniferum*, has been used for medicinal purposes for centuries. Since ancient times, many opiate alkaloids such as morphine have been derived from the poppy plant. In addition, synthetic or semisynthetic opioid agents have been derived by altering the morphine chemical structure. There are three major classes of opioid receptors. Opioids are agents capable of binding opioid receptors and include both natural and synthetic substances.

The classic opioid toxidrome includes central nervous system depression, respiratory depression, and miosis. Other opioid toxic effects include: hypotension, flushing, pruritus, bronchospasm, pulmonary edema, nausea, vomiting, reduced gut motility, and seizures.

The diagnosis of opioid poisoning is a clinical diagnosis. Miosis is often an excellent clue but may be absent in propoxyphene, meperidine, and concurrent co-ingestions. Routine urine drug screening is not required for the diagnosis. Urine drug screening may yield false positives or false negatives as may be the case with synthetic opioids like methadone and propoxyphene. Patient care should be based on clinical presentation and not laboratory diagnostics.

Most deaths related to opioid poisoning are due to respiratory depression and hypoxia. A decrease in tidal volume as well as respiratory rate may be observed in patients who have ingested opioids. Also, there are specific opioid agents that may cause other potentially lethal effects. Propoxyphene may cause cardiac dysrhythmias through effects on myocardial sodium channels. Seizures have been associated with meperidine and tramadol ingestions.

Management of patients with opioid poisoning involves maintenance of airway patency and supportive care. A chest radiograph would be helpful if you suspect aspiration or noncardiogenic pulmonary edema. Naloxone, an opioid receptor antagonist, may be administered to improve respiratory drive and ventilation. Avoid complete reversal of the opioid drug effect to prevent acute withdrawal symptoms in opioid dependent patients. Naloxone can be administered in doses of 0.2–0.4 mg intramuscularly, intravenously, or subcutaneously and titrated to clinical effect. Patients should be observed for re-sedation for 4–6 hours after the last dose of naloxone is given since the half-life of naloxone is shorter than most opioid agents. This observation period should be extended in those patients with renal insufficiency.

Further reading

1 Warner-Smith M, Darke S, Lynskey M, Hall W. Heroin overdose: causes and consequences. *Addiction* 2001;**96**(8):1113–25.
2 Sporer KA. Acute heroin overdose. *Ann Intern Med* 1999; **130**(7):584–90.

Case 82 | Weakness and bradycardia in an elderly female patient

Answer: A
Diagnosis: Third-degree atrioventricular block (AVB)
Discussion: The rhythm strip on page 52 demonstrates complete independent activity of atria and ventricles; furthermore, the atrial and ventricular rhythms are both regular

with a wide QRS complex. These findings are consistent with complete atrioventricular (AV) dissociation, also known as third-degree AVB.

Heart block is a descriptive term used to characterize a disturbance in the conduction of the electrical impulse in the heart – in this case, in and around the AV node. This disturbance can be partial or complete, resulting in either a delayed or an entirely blocked impulse. In complete heart block, no atrial impulses reach the ventricle through the AV node and intraventricular conduction system. The atria and ventricles are functioning independently with control by different pacemakers. The atrial pacemaker can be either sinus or ectopic with a non-sinus focus at normal, slow, or rapid rates. The ventricular rhythm, in essence an escape rhythm, can also have varying pacemaker sites resulting in differing rates; most often, the QRS complexes are regular. The site of ventricular escape rhythm will be immediately below the level of the block. When the ventricular escape rhythm is located near the His bundle, the rate is greater than 40 bpm and the QRS complexes tend to be narrow. When the site of escape is distal to the His bundle, the rate tends to be less than 40 bpm and the QRS complexes tend to be wide, as seen in this case.

In children, the most common cause of third-degree AVB is congenital pathology. In adults, acute coronary syndrome, medication toxicity, and degenerative processes are the most common causes of complete heart block; in fact, acute myocardial infarction is the most frequent etiology of third-degree AVB. Patients with anterior wall acute myocardial infarction (AMI) complicated by third-degree AVB are likely to be significantly compromised by the bradydysrhythmia. The pathophysiology in this setting likely involves irreversible ischemic injury (i.e. infarction) to the intraventricular conduction system. Because the conduction system injury is both permanent and infra-Hisian, medical therapies are unlikely to produce benefit; the response to therapy short of transvenous pacing is limited – these patients should be considered for a transvenous pacing wire and, ultimately, for permanent pacemaker insertion.

Conversely, patients with inferior wall AMI tolerate the block to a greater extent. The ventricular response is usually greater with rates greater than 40 bpm seen in most instances. The site of block is higher in the conduction system – either within the AV node or the His bundle; reversible ischemia to the conduction system complicated by a heightened parasympathetic tone is seen in these patients. If the ventricular rate is greater than 40 bpm and the patient is stable, one can elect to place a transvenous pacer only if the clinical situation deteriorates. If the patient deteriorates, then transvenous pacing should be initiated.

The prediction of third-degree heart block in the ACS patient remains a significant clinical challenge. One useful method to predict this complication considers the presence of the following electrocardiographic findings, including first-degree AVB, second-degree (types I and II) AVB, right bundle branch block (BBB), left BBB, left anterior fascicular block, and left posterior fascicular block. Each risk factor, if present on the electrocardiogram in the setting of an acute coronary syndrome event, is given a score of 1. The total score is then calculated and translated to the rate of occurrence of such third-degree AVB: 0 with a 1.2% risk, 1 with a 7.8% risk, 2 with a 25% risk, and a score of 3 or more with a 36.4% risk.

Further reading

1 Brady WJ, Swart G, DeBehnke DJ, *et al.* The efficacy of atropine in the treatment of hemodynamically unstable bradycardia and atrioventricular block: prehospital and emergency department considerations. *Resuscitation* 1999;**41**:47–55.

2 Lamas FA, Muller JE, Turi ZG, *et al.* A simplified method to predict occurrence of complete heart block during acute myocardial infarction. *Am J Cardiol* 1986;**57**:1213–19.

Case 83 | **Blurred vision following yard work**

Answer: E

Diagnosis: Jimson weed exposure

Discussion: Found throughout North America, jimson weed, *Datura stramonium*, is a tall plant with trumpet-shaped white or violet flowers and bears a seed-containing fruit. Up to 50–100 seeds may be contained in each fruit. All parts of the plant contain parasympatholytic alkaloids including atropine, hyoscamine, and scopolamine, with the highest concentration present in the seeds. One hundred seeds contain the equivalent amount of 6 mg of atropine. Purposeful ingestion of jimson weed is usually for its hallucinogenic effect. Means of ingestion usually involve eating the leaves, pods, or seeds or smoking the leaves and stems. Health hazards arise from behavioral difficulties secondary to the central anticholinergic effects.

Parasympatholytic alkaloids, like those contained in jimson weed, may also cause mydriasis through direct body contact. Unilateral mydriasis is a pharmacologic effect that can occur from direct chemical instillation into the eye or from hand-eye transmission after handling the parasympatholytic agent. Unilateral mydriasis can also occur following ocular exposure to nebulized anticholinergic solution used for respiratory distress.

The emergency physician must consider a broad differential diagnosis for the non-traumatic fixed and dilated pupil, including physiologic anisocoria, third cranial nerve palsy, pharmacologic blockade, and a tonic (Adie) pupil. To differentiate between pharmacologic mydriasis and a third nerve palsy, 1% pilocarpine can be instilled in the mydriatic pupil. A dilated pupil secondary to third nerve injury will respond to pilocarpine by constricting. In the presence of parasympatholytic alkaloids, competitive antagonism of pilocarpine occurs, and the pupil will not constrict (exceptions may occur with ocular trauma or increased intraocular pressure).

Additional work-up of presenting anisocoria should be mandated by the clinical context of the physical findings.

Further reading

1 Tiongson J, Salen P. Mass ingestion of Jimson Weed by eleven teenagers. *Del Med J* 1998;**70**:471–6.
2 Havelius U, Asman P. Accidental mydriasis from exposure to Angel's Trumpet (*Datura suaveolens*). *Acta Ophthalmol Scand* 2002;**80**:332–5.

Case 84 | **A gagging child**

Answer: D

Diagnosis: Esophageal foreign body

Discussion: Evaluation of patients who have ingested foreign bodies is not an uncommon occurrence in the emergency department. Children aged 18–48 months are most likely to swallow solid objects such as toys, coins, pins, and button batteries. Many of these objects are radioopaque and can be seen on plain radiograph. If an ingested foreign body is suspected, plain X-rays of the entire gastrointestinal tract, from neck to anus, are the most appropriate initial imaging study. Many children with impacted esophageal foreign bodies will be asymptomatic, but others may present with drooling, odynophagia, vomiting, and anorexia. These radiographs should be done using a portable X-ray if transport outside the emergency department will put the patient at risk.

Esophageal foreign bodies can be distinguished from those that become trapped in the trachea based on their position on plain radiograph. Due to the ring structure of the trachea, coin shaped or other flat-sided objects tend to lie in the sagittal plane, pushing against the muscular posterior wall of the trachea and are thus seen lying flat on antero-posterior (AP) films. Conversely, objects lodged in the esophagus tend to become lodged in the coronal plane and are therefore seen lying vertically on an AP film and posterior to the tracheal air column on lateral chest radiographs.

Direct visualization of the foreign body by endoscopy is both the diagnostic and therapeutic modality of choice and should be employed emergently for sharp foreign bodies in the esophagus and stomach as well as for ingested button batteries in the esophagus which can cause mucosal necrosis and perforation within hours of impaction. Sharp objects located distal to the pyloric sphincter require emergent surgical consultation.

When plain films fail to identify an ingested foreign body and a high index of suspicion remains, a number of diagnostic options are available. A swallowing study with contrast material may reveal filling defects in the esophagus suggesting the location of a foreign body. This option is limited if there is a high risk for aspiration or if perforation is suspected. Furthermore, any use of contrast materials may complicate endoscopic evaluation. Non-contrast CT scan is excellent for visualizing radiolucent foreign bodies and characterizing other pathology related to longstanding impaction.

In adults, ingested foreign bodies tend to lodge in the lower esophageal sphincter while in children blunt objects can lodge at three anatomic narrowings in the esophagus. The most common site, accounting for approximately 70% of impactions, is the thoracic inlet located between the clavicles on a chest X ray, where the cricopharyngeus muscle acts as a sling to catch these objects. The remaining 30% occur at the level of the aortic arch or the lower esophageal sphincter. If a foreign body is lodged at any other point in the esophagus, underlying esophageal pathology must be suspected. Sharp objects can become lodged at any point along the gastrointestinal tract.

Most foreign bodies will pass spontaneously through the gastrointestinal system, but it must be assumed that a foreign body in the esophagus is impacted and therefore requires intervention. The longer a foreign body remains impacted, the greater risk for complications such as pressure necrosis, infection, stricture formation, and perforation. Once an object has passed into the stomach, it is likely to pass through the rest of the gastrointestinal tract unless it is too long (>6 cm) or too wide (>2 cm) to pass through the pyloric sphincter. Another potential site of impaction is the ileocecal valve.

Several other methods for dislodging blunt esophageal foreign bodies have been described but should be used with caution. One involves the use of a foley catheter passed distal to the level of the foreign body. The foley balloon is then filled with contrast material and both the foley and foreign body are withdrawn under fluoroscopy up the esophagus and out the oropharynx. Another technique involves using a bougie to push an impacted object distally into the stomach, where it will ideally transit the rest of the gastrointestinal tract uneventfully. A third option for objects located in the distal esophagus involves the use of agents such as glucagon and nifedipine that relax the lower esophageal sphincter with expectant passage of the foreign body beyond that point. Emetics (ipecac) are not recommended because of the potential for both aspiration and esophageal injury in the setting of vomiting against a fixed obstruction.

Further reading

1 Kay M, Wyllie R. Pediatric foreign bodies and their management. *Curr Gastroenterol Rep* 2005;**7**(3):212–18.
2 Cheng W, Tam PK. Foreign body ingestion in children: experience with 1265 cases. *J Ped Surg* 1999;**34**(10):1472–6.

Case 85 | A child with bruises of different ages

Answer: B

Diagnosis: Child abuse

Discussion: Much effort has been directed toward collecting information about patterns of bruising in the physical exam of a child in order to allay or corroborate the suspicion of child abuse. This remains an area of active research. Any concern based on bruising alone should always be examined in the context of the developmental status of the child, the clinical scenario, and the explanation given by caregivers (and the consistency of that explanation). While each child should be evaluated in such context, review of the recent medical literature does support the finding that some patterns of bruising are more suggestive of abuse and should therefore alert the physician to consider that possibility.

Some patterns of bruising are more often found with accidental mechanisms and may be more reassuring. For example, bruising of the shins and knees in a child old enough to ambulate independently can be expected as developmentally appropriate. Bruises over bony prominences (e.g., forehead) may also be less suspicious in appropriately mobile children.

In contrast, bruising in a child or infant that is not independently mobile is worthy of some suspicion as the mechanism of falling accidentally is not plausible. There are certain areas of the body, where if bruising is found, abuse may be suggested. These include the face, trunk, arms, hands, and buttocks. If the bruising being examined is located away from bony prominences, it may also deserve scrutiny. Multiple bruising in clusters or with pathognomonic patterns also should be investigated. Examples of the latter might include bruises in a pediatric patient with distinctive imprints (such as from implements like an electrical cord or leather belt) or uniformity of size.

Finally, there is also the issue of estimating the age of bruises. Despite statements in some sources that aging of bruises can be done based on color, a recent review of the existing medical literature has questioned this opinion. No convincing scientific data could be found by the authors of this review to suggest color variation can be used to accurately age a bruise. This review of the literature also found that a clinician's ability to identify the age of a bruise within 24 hours of its creation was poor. Significant intra-observer and inter-observer variability was also reported in these circumstances.

Further reading

1 Maguire S, Mann MK, Sibert J, Kemp A. Are there patterns of bruising in childhood which are diagnostic or suggestive of abuse? A systematic review. *Arch Dis Child* 2005;**90**(2):182–6.
2 Maguire S, Mann MK, Sibert J, Kemp A. Can you age bruises accurately in children? A systematic review. *Arch Dis Child* 2005; **90**(2):187–9.

Case 86 | Traumatic eye pain and proptosis

Answer: E

Diagnosis: Acute retrobulbar hemorrhage

Discussion: Acute retrobulbar hemorrhage can cause severe permanent vision loss if not recognized and treated in the emergency department. Vision loss occurs as the hemorrhage fills the retrobulbar space and transmits pressure on the outside of the globe causing dramatic elevation in the intraocular pressure. The acute rise in pressure can compress the circulation from mechanical tamponade and restrict flow through the central retinal artery. Treatment to lower the intraocular pressure should be initiated immediately when vision is threatened.

Medical treatment for elevated intraocular pressure should be initiated with a topical beta blocker (timolol or levobunolol 0.5%) and alpha agonist (brimonidine 0.15%), one drop each every 30 minutes for two doses. In addition, a carbonic anhydrase inhibitor such as acetazolamide (i.e. two 250 mg tablets orally or 500 mg intravenously) should be given. Mannitol (20%, 1.0 g/kg intravenous) can also decrease intraocular pressure by reducing vitreous volume. Caution must be observed when giving mannitol to patients with congestive heart failure or renal failure.

Performing a lateral canthotomy and cantholysis immediately lowers the intraocular pressure by expanding the intraorbital volume. This is accomplished by first anesthetizing the skin using 2% lidocaine with epinephrine. Next, an incision is made at the lateral canthus exposing the canthal tendons. The lower limb of the canthal tendon is then incised using sharp scissors, releasing the lower lid from its lateral attachment. Surgical repair of the canthotomy/cantholysis is performed several days later when the swelling has subsided. Ophthalmology consultation is required for follow-up.

Further reading

1 Ghufoor K, Sandhu G, Sutcliffe J. Delayed onset of retrobulbar haemorrhage following severe head injury: a case report and review. *Injury* 1998;**29**(2):139–41.
2 Larian B, Wong B, Crumley RL, *et al*. Facial trauma and ocular/orbital injury. *J Craniomaxillofac Trauma* 1999;**5**(4):15–24.

Case 87 | Post-prandial abdominal pain in an elderly woman

Answer: B

Diagnosis: Gallstone ileus with pneumobilia

Discussion: Gallstone ileus is a condition that occurs when a gallstone erodes through the gallbladder wall into adjacent bowel, creating a cholecystoenteric fistula that provides a pathway for gallstones to travel into the duodenum or transverse colon. When large gallstones (>2 cm) travel to a narrow part of the small bowel (distal ileum or jejunum), they can create a mechanical partial obstruction. Although up to one-third of patients with gallstone ileus do not have a history of biliary colic. It typically presents as a small bowel obstruction and is more prevalent in females and the elderly. Gallstone ileus causes almost 25% of all partial small bowel obstructions in patients over 65. Initial plain radiographs will show partial small bowel obstruction in 70% of the cases, but pneumobilia or calcified mass in distal small bowel can be seen in only a third of plain radiographs. Ultrasound can make a definitive diagnosis with the presence of pneumobilia and the detection of the calculus by tracing the dilated small bowel to the site of the obstruction; however, overlying small loops of bowel can obscure deep calculi, and gas within the gallbladder fossa is frequently not recognized. Due to the multitude of causes for small bowel obstruction and the importance of assessing the level and severity of the obstruction, abdomen CT scan with intravenous and oral contrast has been utilized recently to investigate causes for small bowel obstruction.

The presence of gas within the liver must be differentiated by location, either biliary or portal venous system. Portal venous gas tends to be more peripheral and fragmented. The differential diagnosis for portal venous gas includes necrotizing enterocolitis and bowel ischemia. Biliary gas typically outlines the common bile duct and its major branches, and it should prompt one to look for the few causes of pneumobilia: (1) recent surgery (i.e. endoscopic retrograde cholangiopancreatography with sphincterotomy); (2) infection (emphysematous cholecystitis); (3) passage of a gallstone; and (4) the presence of a fistula (cholecystoduodenal or cholecystocolic). When an abdominal CT study reveals the criteria for *Rigler's Triad* of gallstone ileus (small bowel obstruction, pneumobilia, and calcified gallstone in distal small bowel), surgery should be contacted immediately for emergent surgical intervention.

Further reading

1 Reisner RM, Cohen JR. Gallstone ileus: a review of 1001 reported cases. *Am Surg* 1994;**60**(6):441–6.
2 Rivadeneira DE, Curry WT. Images of interest – gastrointestinal: gallstone ileus. *J Gastroenterol Hepatol* 1994;**16**:105.
3 Swift SE, Spencer JA. Gallstone Ileus: CT findings. *Clin Radiol* 1998;**53**:451–4.

Case 88 | Hyperthermia, tachycardia, and confusion in a teenager

Answer: B

Diagnosis: Body packer with cocaine toxicity secondary to packet rupture

Discussion: The plastic bag contains multiple condom wrapped packets of cocaine. This patient is a "body packer," a person who ingests and transports packets of illicit drugs across country lines in order to evade customs officials. This should not to be confused with a "body stuffer," a person who quickly ingests illicit drugs (typically wrapped) to avoid detection by law enforcement officials.

This person demonstrates a sympathomimetic syndrome. On further questioning, this patient stated that he was transporting packets of cocaine from Columbia to the United States. Beta-adrenergic antagonists, including mixed alpha- and

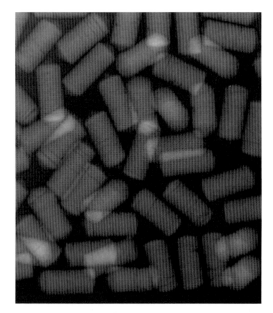

Figure 88.1 An X-ray of the bag of packets noted in the case. Taking a radiograph of the packets, if available, may help to demonstrate their appearance and assist with locating them on a body packer's abdominal radiograph.

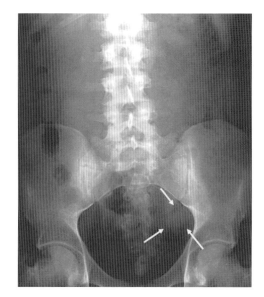

Figure 88.2 The abdominal radiograph from the case with arrows delineating a retained packet near the rectum. This film demonstrates the potential difficulty in localizing drug packets on plain X-ray.

beta-adrenergic antagonists, are contraindicated in cocaine toxicity. Beta-blockers can potentially induce unopposed alpha agonist activity, placing the patients at risk for vasospasm. The patient should be treated with benzodiazepines, such as lorazepam, in an attempt to decrease his sympathomimetic state. Benzodiazepines should be titrated until the patient has calmed and his heart rate has diminished, which may take larger than typical doses. If marked hypertension persists despite benzodiazepines, nitrates, and phentolamine can be utilized.

In the asymptomatic packer, gastrointestinal decontamination with activated charcoal concurrently with polyethylene glycol is the mainstay of decreasing potential drug absorption and decreasing enteric transit time until rectal elimination.

If the patient were to develop cardiac dysrhythmias, sodium channel blocking agents such as procainamide should be avoided in cocaine toxicity. Cocaine is itself a cardiac sodium channel blocker. If QRS prolongation or cardiac dysrhythmias developed, sodium bicarbonate should be the pharmacologic treatment administered first.

Further reading

1 Traub SJ, Hoffman RS, Nelson LS. Body packing – the internal concealment of illicit drugs. *New Engl J Med* 2003;**349**(26):2519–26.
2 Beno S, Calello D, Baluffi A, Henretig FM. Pediatric body packing: drug smuggling reaches a new low. *Pediatr Emerg Care* 2005; **21**(11):744–6.

Case 89 | **Acute onset double vision**

Answer: C
Diagnosis: Third cranial nerve palsy
Discussion: This patient has an isolated, pupil-involving third nerve palsy of the left eye. The third cranial nerve innervates the superior, inferior, and medial recti muscles as well as the inferior oblique muscle. In addition, parasympathetic fibers to the pupillary sphincter muscle run along the dorsal and peripheral aspect of the third cranial nerve. Patients with third

nerve dysfunction typically present with a ptosis, limited ocular motility, and variable pupil involvement.

Isolated third nerve palsy with pupillary involvement must be presumed secondary to an aneurysm until proven otherwise. The most common site is at the junction of the posterior communicating artery and the internal carotid artery. A magnetic resonance imaging (MRI) with contrast and magnetic resonance angiography (MRA) should be obtained emergently.

Isolated pupil-sparing third nerve palsy implies complete loss of ocular motility with normal pupillary function. These palsies presumably result from microvascular injury and are most often seen in older patients with hypertension or diabetes. Neuroimaging is not necessary in patients over 50 years of age if vasculopathic risk factors are present. These typically resolve spontaneously over 2–3 months.

Pain is not helpful in determining the etiology of a third nerve palsy. Even though most patients with aneurysmal third nerve palsies complain of pain, many microvascular third nerve palsies also present with pain. Neuro-ophthalmology or neurology consult is warranted for patients presenting to the emergency department with a third nerve palsy.

Further reading

1 Lee AG, Hayman LA, Brazis PW. The evaluation of isolated third nerve palsy revisited: an update on the evolving role of magnetic resonance, computed tomography, and catheter angiography. *Surv Ophthalmol* 2002;**47**(2):137–57.

2 Bennett JL, Pelak VS. Palsies of the third, fourth, and sixth cranial nerves. *Ophthalmol Clin North Am* 2001;**14**(1): 169–85.

Case 90 | **Ankle pain and inability to walk**

Answer: D

Diagnosis: Trimalleolar fracture

Discussion: Ankle fractures and dislocations are among the most common orthopedic injuries cared for in the emergency department. The majority of ankle injuries involve a rotational mechanism. Patients typically report immediate onset of pain following the traumatic event and inability to bear weight.

The initial evaluation of a patient with an acute ankle injury begins with a directed history. The mechanism of the injury will focus the evaluation toward understood patterns of injury. Information regarding the patient's ability to ambulate following the event assists in the decision to obtain radiographs. Secondary injuries from the traumatic event and the cause of the event should be identified. A directed physical exam is performed to identify areas of tenderness. The ankle joint includes the distal fibula, tibia and the talus. Examination of the knee and foot is necessary to evaluate for secondary injuries associated with ankle injury (fractures of the proximal fibula and base of the fifth metatarsal in particular). The bony structures of the ankle are easily palpable secondary to minimal soft-tissue coverage. Careful examination of the medial ankle includes assessing for tenderness of the distal tibia and the deltoid ligament. Examination of the lateral ankle includes assessment of the distal fibula and the anterior talofibular, posterior talofibular, and calcaneofibular ligaments. The anterior ankle is palpated to assess for injury to the tibiofibular syndesmotic ligament and the Achilles tendon is palpated in the posterior ankle. Neurovascular status is examined to exclude secondary injury.

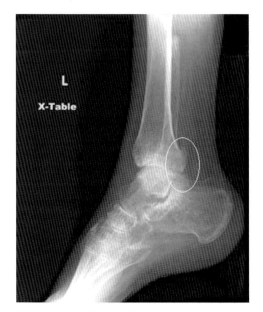

Figure 90.1 Lateral ankle view demonstrates fracture of the posterior malleolus of the tibia (circle).

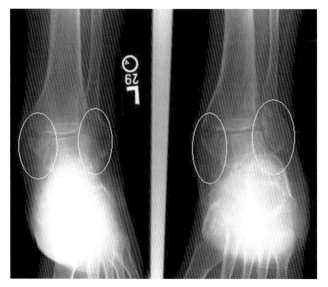

Figure 90.2 AP ankle radiograph demonstrates displaced fracture of the distal tibia at the level of the talar dome. An oblique fracture of the distal fibula is visualized. Both fractures are also apparent on the mortise view. Fractures are noted by a circle annotation.

The decision to perform radiographs can be guided by the Ottawa Ankle rules (OAR). Following the OARs, radiographs are obtained if there is an inability to bear weight immediately after the event or in the emergency department (ED), or if there is tenderness at the tip or posterior aspect of the distal 6 cm of the medial or lateral malleolus. Anteroposterior (AP) and lateral radiographs will reveal the majority of ankle fractures. Additionally, the mortise view (AP rotated 15 degrees internally) may be of assistance if suspicion for bony injury is high and standard views are equivocal.

Fractures of the ankle joint are classified either as stable or unstable. Stable fractures involve one side of the ankle joint, either the medial or lateral malleolus. If the fracture involves either malleolus with ligamentous disruption of the opposite side of the ankle, the fracture is identified as unstable. An example is a fracture of the lateral malleolus and disruption of the medial deltoid ligament.

Unstable ankle fractures involve both sides of the ankle joint. They can be further classified as a bimalleolar fracture (involvement of the medial and lateral malleoli) or trimalleolar fracture (involvement of the posterior, medial and lateral malleoli). A trimalleolar fracture is apparent in this case.

Treatment of an unstable ankle fracture involves open reduction and internal fixation. The articular cartilage of the ankle requires proper alignment as small deviations lead to significant risk of posttraumatic arthritic changes. Precise alignment is best achieved operatively. The timing of surgery is dependent on multiple clinical factors including patient stability, secondary injuries, and co-morbidities. Orthopedic consultation should be obtained after the identification of the fracture for operative planning.

Further reading

1 Kay RM, Matthys GA. Pediatric ankle fractures: evaluation and treatment. *J Am Acad Orthopedic Surg* 2001;**9**:268.
2 Deasy C, Murphy D, McMahon GC, Kelly IP. Ankle fractures: emergency department management… is there room for improvement? *Eur J Emerg Med* 2005;**12**(5): 216–19.
3 DeVries JS, Wijgman AJ, Sierevelt IN, Schaap GR. Long-term results of ankle fractures with a posterior malleolar fragment. *J Foot Ankle Surg* 2005;**44**(3):211–17.

Case 91 | Tongue swelling in a hypertensive female

Answer: C

Diagnosis: Angioedema secondary to angiotensin converting enzyme inhibitor (ACEI)

Discussion: Angioedema is a condition marked by nondependent, asymmetric, non-pitting edema that results from a loss of vascular integrity and extravasation of fluid into the interstitial tissues of the body with preference for the face, lips, tongue, oropharynx, and larynx. Two distinct mechanisms, mast cell-mediated and non-mast cell-mediated angioedema (MCMA and NMCMA), have been implicated in the majority of case presentations.

MCMA can be viewed as an extension of the more superficial process of urticaria formation. Whereas the edema associated with urticaria is confined to the superficial dermis, MCMA involves edema formation in the deep dermis and subdermal tissues. This process is mediated by the release of histamine, leukotrienes, and prostaglandins from mast cells causing increased vasodilation and capillary permeability with resultant edema formation. Typical causes of MCMA include food and drug exposures. Chronic cases have been linked to an autoimmune process whereby antibodies directly activate mast cells. Treatment of MCMA begins with cessation of any offending agent. Additionally, antihistamines and corticosteroids are useful. Epinephrine remains the treatment of choice for any airway compromise or vasomotor instability. A defining feature of MCMA is its association with the presence of urticaria and/or pruritus in 90% of cases. The absence of

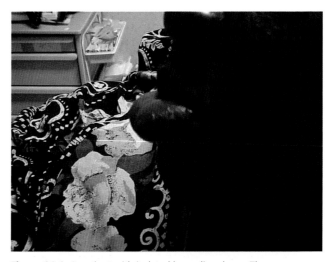

Figure 91.1 A patient with isolated lower lip edema. The cause was found to be secondary to her ACEI (missed on her first presentation to the emergency department 1 week previously). This swelling resolved after 4 hours of observation in the emergency department. No pharmacologic therapy was necessary.

these symptoms should prompt the clinician to consider causes of NMCMA.

NMCMA occurs in the absence of urticaria and pruritus and is thought to occur independently of mast cell degranulation. Two proposed mechanisms for the development of NMCMA include increased activity of bradykinin and abnormalities in the complement cascade (i.e. C1-esterase inhibitor deficiency). The most common cause of NMCMA presenting to emergency rooms is exposure to ACEI. NMCMA occurs in 0.1–0.7% of patients taking ACEI and is more common in older patients and African-Americans. NMCMA from ACEI use typically occurs within days to weeks after therapy is started, but can develop years after uneventful use. ACEI induced NMCMA is not related to the development of ACEI induced cough and has equal likelihood of development with all ACEI.

Bradykinin is a potent vasodilator that normally functions to oppose the vasoconstrictive effects of angiotensin II. Angiotensin converting enzyme functions to increase production of angiotensin II and decrease the activity of bradykinin. The antihypertensive effects of ACEI therefore become apparent, causing a relative decrease in angiotensin II (decreased vasoconstriction) and a relative increase in bradykinin activity (increased vasodilation). It is this rise in bradykinin activity that is thought to be responsible for the (NMCMA) associated with ACEI use.

Treatment of NMCMA requires particular focus on the patient's airway and vasomotor stability. Epinephrine (0.3–0.5 mg intramuscular) and definitive airway management (endotracheal intubation or surgical airway) are required for any airway or circulatory compromise. Antihistamines and corticosteroids may have some benefit and their administration should be considered in patients with NMCMA.

NMCMA related to a deficiency in the C1-esterase inhibitor, a component of the complement cascade, occurs in both hereditary (hereditary angioedema or HAE) and acquired forms. HAE typically presents in childhood following traumatic or stressful situations, while the acquired form is commonly associated with certain malignancies and presents at an older age. This form of angioedema is treated in the acute setting in identical fashion as ACEI induced NMCMA. In addition, androgens (stanozol 2–4 mg/day and danazol 200–400 mg/day) have been used to treat this condition both prophylactically and in the acute setting. Fresh frozen plasma has been given to acutely replete the C1-esterase inhibitor protein.

Further reading

1 Baxi S, Dinakar C. Urticaria and angioedema. *Immunol Allergy Clin North Am* 2005;**25**(2):353–67.
2 Hide M, Francis DM, Grattan CE, *et al.* Autoantibioties against the high affinity IgE receptor as a cause of histamine release in chronic urticaria. *New Engl J Med* 1993; **328**:1599–604.
3 Brown NJ, Ray WA, Snowden M, Griffin MR. Black Americans have an increased rate of angiotensin enzyme inhibitor-associated angioedema. *Cli Pharmacol Ther* 1996;**60**:8–13.

Case 92 | **Wide complex tachycardia in an older male patient**

Answer: C

Diagnosis: Wide complex tachycardia – ventricular tachycardia

Discussion: The two electrocardiographic rhythm strips in this case (lead II and the V lead) demonstrate a wide QRS complex tachycardia (WCT). The QRS complex is markedly wide with a very rapid, regular rhythm. There is also the presence of atrioventricular (AV) dissociation in lead II (Figure 92.1, arrows), which is very strongly suggestive of ventricular tachycardia (VT) as the rhythm diagnosis.

A WCT is defined electrocardiographically as a dysrhythmia with a QRS complex greater than 0.12 second in duration and a ventricular rate greater than 120 bpm. In patients presenting with a WCT, the differentiation of VT from supraventricular tachycardia (SVT) with aberrant ventricular conduction is difficult. Aberrant ventricular conduction may be due to a pre-existing bundle branch block (BBB), a functional (rate-related) bundle malfunction resulting in a widened QRS complex when the heart rate exceeds a characteristic maximum for that patient, or accessory AV conduction as encountered in pre-excitation syndromes (Wolff–Parkinson–White syndrome).

Certain clinical variables may support a diagnosis of VT in the WCT presentation. Patient age greater than 50 years suggests VT; younger age is associated with SVT yet in a less robust fashion. Consideration of the past medical history also is helpful; a history of angina, myocardial infarction, coronary artery bypass grafting, valvular heart disease, or congestive heart failure strongly suggests VT. It must be stressed that the presence or absence of hemodynamic instability does not support either diagnosis; either dysrhythmia can present with instability or stability.

Electrocardiographic variables suggestive of VT (Figure 92.2) include a broad QRS complex, AV dissociation, fusion beats, capture beats, and QRS complex features. When noted, AV dissociation is diagnostic of VT; unfortunately, AV dissociation is uncommon and, if present, difficult to discern. The second useful feature in establishing a diagnosis of VT is the presence of fusion (a combination of a supraventricular impulse with a ventricular impulse, producing a QRS complex of different morphology) or capture (a supraventricular impulse passes through the AV node, causing an electrical depolarization of the ventricles) beats; the finding of either a fusion or a capture beat confirms the diagnosis of VT, but

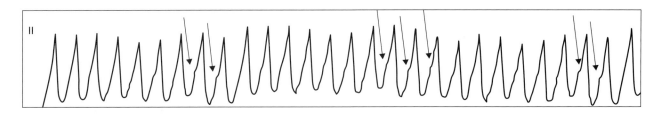

Figure 92.1 The presence of AV dissociation in lead II (arrows) is very strongly suggestive of VT as the rhythm diagnosis.

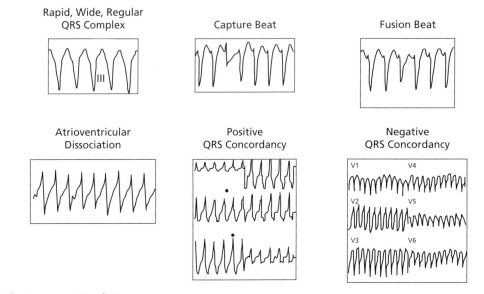

Figure 92.2 ECG features suggestive of VT.

again its utility is limited. Fusion and/or capture beats are observed in less than 10% of cases of VT. QRS complex concordance (precordial QRS complexes entirely positive or negative) favors VT.

The limited usefulness of these features has led to the construction of several stepwise approaches to the diagnosis of WCT. For example, the approach suggested by Brugada and Brugada involves a four-step algorithm. This tool, as well as numerous similar proposals, however, is somewhat cumbersome. Also, the majority of these protocols have a default diagnosis of SVT with aberration. Clearly, defaulting to a less severe diagnosis is problematic, fraught with error and danger for the patient and clinician. Certainly, the clinician is required to treat the patient – not the electrocardiogram (ECG). In other words,

with the idea that the specific rhythm diagnosis may not be possible, the clinician should focus on the patient and his/her hemodynamic status – and base initial therapy on the entire clinical picture; furthermore, the clinician should not default to a less severe illness – SVT with aberration; if in doubt, manage the patient as if VT is the rhythm diagnosis.

Further reading

1 Hudson KB, Brady WJ, Chan TC, Pollack M, Harrigan RA. Electrocardiographic features of ventricular tachycardia. *J Emerg Med* 2003;**25**:303–14.
2 Brugada P, Brugada J, Mont L, Smeets J, Andries EW. A new approach to the differential diagnosis of a regular tachycardia with a wide QRS complex. *Circulation* 1991;**83**:1649–59.

Case 93 | **Acute onset double vision**

Answer: E
Diagnosis: Ocular foreign body

Discussion: Ocular foreign bodies are frequently encountered in emergency departments. The evaluation of patients presenting with possible ocular foreign bodies is dictated by a careful history. The mechanism of injury and suspected particulate matter is crucial in determining the presence and location of the foreign body. For instance, a history of metal striking metal should raise concern for possible intraocular foreign body. Visual acuity must be documented prior to examining the eye or performing any procedure. Perform a careful pupillary evaluation with attention to the size and shape of each pupil as well as response to stimulation. Thorough slit lamp examination should be conducted for any irregularities or asymmetry in the conjunctiva, cornea, anterior chamber, iris, or lens. The eyelids must be everted, provided there is no evidence of globe perforation, when a foreign body is suspected under the lids. Dilated fundus examination is required for patients with suspected intraocular foreign body. Ultrasound or CT scan of the orbits may be necessary when an intraocular or intraorbital foreign body is suspected.

The photos at the foot of the page show the corneal foreign body of the case presented before and after removal. The photo on the right reveals a residual rust ring and corneal infiltrate. Corneal foreign bodies are best evaluated with a slit lamp. Assessment of the foreign body depth should be determined prior to removal. Foreign bodies that have penetrated into the anterior chamber should be removed in the operating room. Most embedded foreign bodies can be removed at the slit lamp

under topical anesthesia using a 25 g needle or foreign body spud. A red-brown rust ring results if a foreign body has been embedded for more than a few hours. The rust ring is best removed using a battery-powered ophthalmic burr. Therapy following a foreign body removal includes a broad-spectrum antibiotic. Cycloplegia should be considered if an anterior chamber reaction is present. Reexamination in 24 hours is required.

The photograph below left demonstrates an everted eyelid with an insect stuck to the palpebral conjunctiva. Vertical linear scratches on the cornea often indicate a foreign body embedded in the palpebral conjunctiva under the eyelid. The linear scratches result from the foreign body rubbing on the cornea as the patient blinks their eyes. Conjunctival foreign bodies can usually be removed with a moist cotton-tip applicator or simple irrigation. A broad-spectrum antibiotic ointment should be instilled after foreign body removal.

The pictures at the top of the page 144 demonstrate a defect near the pupillary border (white arrow); dilated exam reveals a posterior subcapsular cataract with an intraocular foreign body imbedded in the posterior lens (red arrow). The diagnosis of a penetrating ocular injury is often obvious to the observer; however, some may be quite subtle and require a high index of suspicion and careful observation. A detailed history and nature of the injury should be obtained. Visual acuity must be documented and a careful examination performed. Signs suggestive of intraocular foreign body include deep eyelid laceration, conjunctival laceration/hemorrhage, iris-corneal adhesion, shallow anterior chamber, hypotony, iris defect, and acute cataract. A CT scan of the brain and orbits (1 mm axial and coronal views) should be obtained. Since over 90% of intraocular foreign bodies are metallic, MRI is contraindicated in most cases of suspected intraocular foreign body. Patients suspected of having an intraocular foreign body require ophthalmologic consultation. The eye should be protected with a shield. Patients should be NPO and placed on bedrest with bathroom privileges. Tetanus should be given when indicated and antiemetics prescribed to prevent Valsalva.

This patient pictured on page 144 (bottom picture) has suffered a perforating ocular injury with an entrance wound

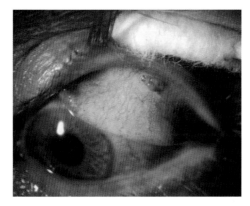

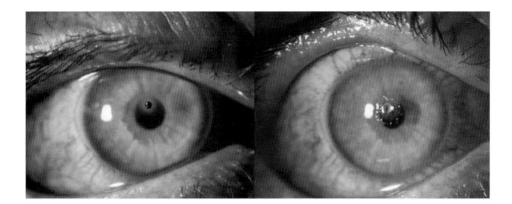

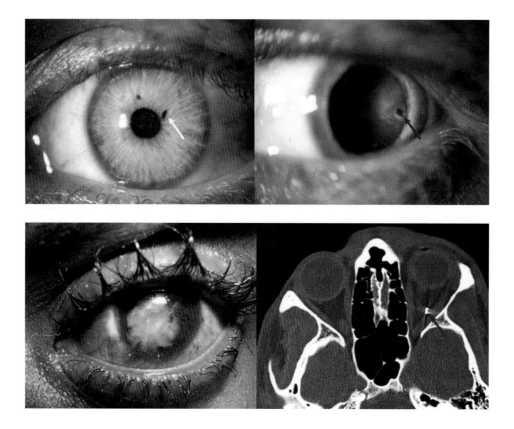

in the cornea and an exit wound somewhere in the posterior pole of the eye. The white substance in the anterior chamber is hydrated lens material that resulted from the foreign body passing through the lens and disrupting the lens capsule. A CT scan of the brain and orbits is indicated for all patients suspected of having an ocular or orbital foreign body. The CT scan in this case shows an intraorbital foreign body (red arrow) in the posterior orbit lodged between the lateral rectus muscle and the optic nerve. The patient also has a positive Seidel test. This is a simple test to determine if a full-thickness wound is present. It is performed using fluorescein and a cobalt blue light. Fluorescein is instilled in the eye and the wound is observed using the blue light. A test is positive when aqueous leaks out of the wound and is seen washing away the fluorescein.

Management of patients with an intraorbital foreign body in the emergency department involves shielding the eye and consulting ophthalmology. Tetanus toxoid should be given when indicated. Hospitalization is necessary for foreign bodies requiring surgical removal. Patients should be treated with a 10–14-day course of systemic antibiotics. Patients should be monitored closely for evidence of infection.

Further reading

1 Mester V, Kuhn F. Intraocular foreign bodies. *Ophthalmol Clin North Am* 2002;**15**(2):235–42.
2 Williams DF, Mieler WF, Abrams GW, Lewis H. Results and prognostic factors in penetrating ocular injuries with retained intraocular foreign bodies. *Ophthalmology* 1988;**95**:911–16.

Case 94 | **Foot pain in a gymnast**

Answer: C
Diagnosis: Dancer's fracture (fracture in the distal shaft of the 5th metatarsal)

Discussion: A fracture of the distal shaft of the 5th metatarsal is commonly referred to as a "dancer's fracture" because of its association with ballet dancers. Dancer's fracture is characterized by a spiral-oblique fracture in the mid-shaft or neck of the 5th metatarsal. In one specific ballet technique (dem pointe maneuver), a high twisting force is applied in the forefoot and can stress the 5th metatarsal enough to cause a fracture. This fracture can also result from direct trauma to the lateral foot. The classic patient presents with a painful limp but can bear weight on the affected foot. The most common physical exam finding is tenderness over 5th metatarsal and swelling over the lateral aspect of the foot. Another common fracture that must be excluded is a Jones fracture (transverse fracture of the proximal diaphysis of the 5th metatarsal). Jones fractures have a significant risk of malunion or nonunion.

Sagittal, mediolateral, and anterioposterior planes of the affected foot must be obtained to assess for angulation and displacement of the distal fragment. Conservative treatment with a short-leg cast or stiff shoe for 2–6 weeks is recommended for most cases. Prolonged nonweight bearing is associated with an increased risk for reflex sympathetic dystrophy. Closed reduction in the emergency department is required for fractures where there is angulation of greater than 10 degrees or a displacement of greater than 3 mm. Due to the conservative management of this injury, special attention must be given to the sagittal plane radiograph to assess for angulation. A healed angulated 5th metatarsal shaft may be complicated by plantar keratosis in the future. Indications for open reduction include: compartment syndrome, unstable or open fractures, or a failed closed reduction. Orthopedic consultation in the emergency department is recommended for multiple or displaced fractures.

Further reading

1 Ankle and Foot. *Rosen's Emergency Medicine Concepts and Clinical Practice.* 5th Ed. Vol. 1, Marx JA, Ed. St. Louis, MO: Mosby. 2002:728–9.

2 O'Malley MJ, Hamilton WG, Munyak J. Fractures of the distal shaft of the fifth metatarsal. Dancer's fracture. *Am J Sport Med* 1996;**24**(2):240–3.

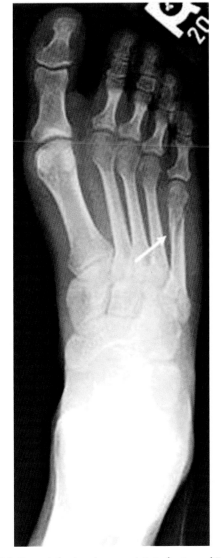

Figure 94.1 Dancer's fracture (arrow points to fracture of 5th metatarsal).

Case 95 | **New facial droop**

Answer: A

Diagnosis: Bell's palsy

Discussion: The patient pictured on page 60 has Bell's palsy. Note ptosis of the left eye and the weakness of the orbicularis muscles on the left side of the face. Also note the absence of wrinkling to the forehead on the affected left side. Bell's palsy is the most common disorder affecting the facial nerve. It is an abrupt, isolated, unilateral, peripheral facial paralysis without detectable causes. While the actual pathophysiology is unknown, the most widely accepted theory postulates inflammation of the facial nerve causing it to be compressed as it courses through the temporal bone.

The incidence in the United States is approximately 23 cases per 100,000 persons. It occurs equally in men and women, most commonly between ages 10 and 40. Clinical conditions associated with Bell's palsy include pregnancy (especially third trimester), immunocompromised states, and diabetes. Patients may present with a concern that they have suffered a stroke. Other common symptoms include pain in or behind the ear, numbness on the affected side of the face, a recent upper respiratory infection, drooling, alteration in taste, and hyperacusis.

The classic definition describes a lower motor neuron deficit of the facial nerve, manifesting as weakness of the entire face (upper and lower) on the affected side. This is in contradistinction to upper motor neuron lesions such as a cortical stroke, where the upper third of the face is spared while the lower two-thirds are paralyzed. While considered an idiopathic facial paralysis, there is significant evidence to support an infectious cause. Herpes simplex virus (HSV-1) has been isolated in many patients and is the most likely infectious agent, although there are likely other etiologic agents with a shared common pathway leading to facial nerve dysfunction.

No specific laboratory tests exist to diagnose Bell's palsy. Clinical suspicion helps to direct what tests may be of value, and may include thyroid function studies and Lyme titer. One can also consider obtaining (if clinically suspected) a rapid plasma reagin (RPR) or a venereal disease research laboratory (VDRL) test for syphilis, as well as a human immunodeficiency virus (HIV) test. There is no evidence to support emergent imaging studies with Bell's palsy.

The primary treatment in the emergency department is with pharmacologic management. The remainder of care focuses on patient education as to the course of the disease and eye care instructions. While considered by some to be controversial, treatment with steroids remains common if the patient presents within 7 days of symptom onset. The postulated mechanism of action is in reducing facial nerve swelling. Current data supports using steroids as a means to improve outcomes, and earlier treatment is preferred (i.e. prednisone at 40–60 mg/day for 7–14 days). Recent evidence supports HSV as the presumed cause in more than 70% of cases; therefore, antiviral agents are a logical choice for pharmacologic management. Recommendations include acyclovir 400–800 mg five times a day for 10 days or valcyclovir 1 g three times a day for 10 days.

The eye on the affected side is potentially at risk for corneal drying and foreign body exposure, as the lid may not close completely, especially when the patient is asleep. This is generally managed with artificial tears and some form of eye protection (patch or glasses during the day, taping the eye shut at night).

The vast majority (85% or more) of patients recover without any cosmetically obvious deformities. Ultimately, 10% will have some residual asymmetry of the facial muscles, and 5% will suffer from significant facial nerve deficits. In most cases, recovery begins 3 weeks after symptom onset, but may take up to a year for complete resolution. Patients with incomplete facial nerve involvement have a more favorable prognosis than those with a complete deficit.

Further reading

1 Gilden DH. Bell's palsy. *New Engl J Med* 2004;**351**(13): 1323–31.
2 Murakami S, Mizobuchi M, Nakashiro Y. Bell palsy and herpes simplex virus: identification of viral DNA in endoneurial fluid and muscle. *Ann Int Med* 1996;**124**:27–30.
3 Ramsey MJ, DerSimonian R, Holtel MR, Burgess LP. Corticosteroid treatment for idiopathic facial nerve paralysis: a meta-analysis. *Laryngoscope* 2000;**110**:335–41.

Case 96 | **Eye pain and swelling**

Answer: A

Diagnosis: Periorbital cellulitis

Discussion: Periorbital cellulitis, also called preseptal cellulitis, is a superficial skin infection which has not penetrated the orbital septum. Its presentation mimics the more serious orbital cellulitis, also called postseptal cellulitis, which is an infection of the deeper tissues of the orbit. In the majority of cases, the distinction can be made clinically without the need for radiographic studies. In cases where the clinical diagnosis is in question, an enhanced CT of the orbits can aid in making a definitive diagnosis.

Periorbital cellulitis in adults and children over 5 years is usually the result of a secondary skin infection with *S. aureus* as the predominant pathogen. In children of 5 years and under, *S. aureus* is still the most common pathogen but *H. influenzae* is responsible for a significant minority, usually from bacteremic spread. Periorbital cellulitis in those of 5 years and older can be treated with oral antibiotics and followed up as outpatients. Children less than 5 years are more likely to have a bacteremic source and should be treated with intravenous antibiotics to cover *S. aureus* and *H. influenzae*, have a blood culture drawn, and should be considered candidates for hospital admission.

Orbital cellulitis is a more serious diagnosis. Figure 96.1 demonstrates a child with orbital cellulitis. This photograph demonstrates proptosis, edema, and limited ocular motility in the right eye as the child looks up to the left.

The majority of orbital cellulitis cases result as an extension from an adjacent bacterial sinusitis. Orbital cellulitis in adults is usually a polymicrobial infection whereas in children it is often caused by a single organism. The differential diagnosis of orbital cellulitis includes preceptal cellulitis, orbital pseudotumor, thyroid eye disease, orbital tumors, metastatic disease, varix, and trauma.

The CT scan in Figure 96.2 demonstrates a subperiosteal abscess (red arrow) overlying a nearly opacified sinus. CT scanning is essential in cases of suspected orbital cellulitis to confirm the diagnosis, to evaluate the sinuses, and to rule

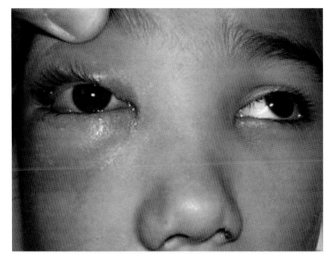

Figure 96.1 Orbital cellulitis.

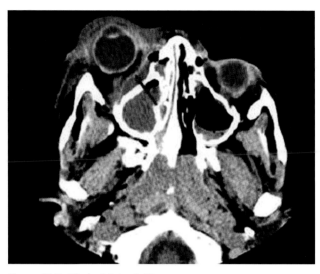

Figure 96.2 CT of orbital cellulitis.

out orbital foreign body. Mucormycosis is a life-threatening disease which must be considered in diabetic and immuno-compromised patients presenting with orbital cellulitis.

Treatment for orbital cellulitis includes admission to the hospital for intravenous antibiotics. Blood cultures should be obtained. ENT should be consulted for surgical drainage if clinically indicated. Patients must be observed closely for optic nerve dysfunction by monitoring visual acuity and pupillary responses.

Periorbital and orbital cellulitis can usually be distinguished on clinical grounds. Periorbital cellulitis presentations typically lack fever and have normal eye examinations, including full range of all extra-ocular eye movements, normal pupillary reflexes, and normal visual acuity. In equivocal cases, CT of the orbits can help make the diagnosis.

Further reading

1 Givner LB. Periorbital versus orbital cellulitis. *Pediatr Infect Dis J* 2002;**21**(12):1157–8.
2 Tovilla-Canales JL, Nava A, Tovilla y Pomar JL. Orbital and peri-orbital infections. *Curr Opin Ophthalmol* 2001; **12**(5):335–41.

Case 97 | **Shortening and rotation of the leg following trauma**

Answer: D

Diagnosis: Left hip fracture

Discussion: This patient has a left hip fracture. Hip fractures include fractures of both the pelvis at the acetabulum and the proximal femur. Fractures of the femoral neck and intertrochanteric fractures cause the classic physical examination findings of the lower extremity seen in this case consisting of foreshortening and external rotation of the lower extremity. While examining the lower extremity, careful attention should be focused to the neurovascular exam.

Fractures of the femoral neck are associated with fractures of the femoral shaft in 20% of patients. A high index of suspicion must be present as the shaft fracture is missed in as many as 40% of patients. The patient's X-ray in this case is noted below.

The X-ray reveals that this patient has sustained an intertrochanteric fracture of the left femur. This injury in younger adults typically occurs after a high-speed motor vehicle crash or a fall from a height. In older patients, this fracture can occur after a fall of any type. A significant force is required to cause this fracture and it is therefore approximately 50% of cases that have other associated injuries.

A complete trauma evaluation must be performed. The patient may be distracted by pain secondary to the hip fracture and unaware of other injuries. Femur fractures can result in the loss of 2–3 units of blood into the thigh and therefore hemodynamic instability can ensue. The patient should have a type and crossmatch sent for at least 2 units of blood. The physician must rule out other potential sources of hemodynamic instability before attributing blood loss to the hip fracture alone. Complete trauma evaluation must be the first priority, then orthopedic consult should be obtained. Internal fixation is usually performed on an urgent, not emergent basis.

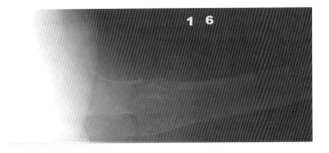

Hip fractures can have a subtle appearance on X-ray. Occult fractures of the hip not seen on X-ray are possible and diagnosis may require magnetic resonance imaging (MRI). There are several radiographic methods to help locate fractures on plain films. One technique is to follow Shenton's line. This is a curved line that extends from the superior border of the obturator foramen down along the medial aspect of the femur. If there is disruption of the smooth C shape that is normally present, fracture or dislocation should be suspected. Another technique is to look for the S and reverse S curves that are present on the medial and lateral aspects of a normal femoral head and neck. If disrupted, the presence of a fracture should be suspected.

Further reading

1 Rudman N, McIlmail D. Emergency department evaluation and treatment of hip and thigh injuries. *Emerg Med Clin North Am* 2000;**18**(1):29–66.
2 Perron AD, Miller MD, Brady WJ. Orthopedic pitfalls in the ED: radiographically occult hip fracture. *Am J Emerg Med* 2002;**20**(3): 234–7.

Case 98 | **Spider bite in the night**

Answer: D

Diagnosis: Black widow envenomation

Discussion: Black widow spiders (*Latrodectus* species) are found over a wide geographic range on every continent but Antarctica. The female spider is responsible for the characteristic toxicity and is shiny black in color with a red hour glass of varying size on its ventral abdomen. Its webs are disorganized, appear abandoned, and are often found near human habitation.

The venom of the black widow contains alpha-latrotoxin. This toxin binds to multiple sites resulting in the unregulated opening of cation channels and the subsequent influx of calcium at presynaptic neurons. Elevated cytosolic calcium causes unregulated release of neurotransmitters. As a result, neurotransmitters, such as acetylcholine and norepinephrine, are increased. This results in activation of both the sympathomimetic and cholinergic systems, and causes increased stimulation at the neuromuscular junction.

Initially, a pinprick sensation may be felt at the bite site. However, the initial pain may go unnoticed. Locally, a small circle of erythema and/or induration may be seen at the bite site. Within the ensuing hours, systemic signs and symptoms may develop, progress, and last for days. Muscle cramping is a characteristic finding associated with black widow envenomation. The cramps may be mild and remain localized to the site or the cramps can involve all muscle groups diffusely and become severe and unrelenting. The worst cases may develop opisthotonus posturing and abdominal rigidity. Nausea, vomiting, headache, palpitations, hypertension, tachycardia, diaphoresis, priapism, facial edema, renal failure, and anxiety may all be clinically seen. The diagnosis of black widow envenomation is made solely on the clinical presentation; there are no clinical laboratory tests available to confirm the diagnosis.

Wounds should be cleansed and if needed tetanus prophylaxis administered. Patients should be monitored for at least 6 hours. In those patients manifesting muscular spasms, opioid analgesics orally or intravenously should be considered. Antispasmodics, such as diazepam, may also provide additional relief. Methocarbamol and dantrolene have been utilized for treatment, with mixed results. Intravenous calcium was initially touted to be efficacious to alleviate the pain associated with cramps, but subsequent studies have not found it to be of significant benefit. Tourniquets have no role in first aid management of black widow envenomations.

Latrodectus mactans antivenom (equine-derived) is rapidly effective at relieving the clinical effects associated with toxicity. However, its use is limited to those patients manifesting significant toxicity not relieved by conventional therapy, or those with health problems that place them at increased risk for complications. The antivenom has an associated risk of anaphylaxis and if utilized, should be administered in a hospitalized setting with full resuscitation capabilities.

Further reading

1 Singletary EM, Rochman AS, Bodmer JC, Holstege CP. Envenomations. *Med Clin North Am* 2005;**89**(6):1195–224.
2 Saucier JR. Arachnid envenomation. *Emerg Med Clin North Am* 2004;**22**:405–22.

Case 99 | **Wide complex tachycardia in a young adult**

Answer: C

Diagnosis: Antidromic tachycardia in Wolff–Parkinson–White syndrome

Discussion: The case rhythm strip demonstrates a wide complex tachycardia (WCT). The electrocardiogram (ECG) reveals the classic electrocardiographic triad of the Wolff–Parkinson–White syndrome (WPW), including shortened PR interval, widened QRS complex, and delta wave.

The WPW syndrome is a form of ventricular pre-excitation involving an accessory conduction pathway. This accessory conduction pathway bypasses the atrioventricular (AV) node, creating a direct electrical connection between the atria and ventricles – in essence, removing the protective, rate-limiting effect of the AV node and subjecting the ventricles to excessive rates when the patient experiences a dysrhythmia. The ventricles are "pre-excited" with atrial impulse conduction over the accessory pathway (AP) which arrives at the ventricular myocardium sooner than the same impulse conducted through the AV node. The electrocardiographic definition of WPW (Figure 99.1) relies on the following electrocardiographic features: (1) a PR interval less than 0.12 seconds; (2) with a slurring of the initial segment of the QRS complex (delta wave); (3) a widened QRS complex; and (4) secondary repolarization changes reflected in ST-segment–T-wave changes. The PR interval is shortened because the impulse progressing down the AP is not subjected to the physiological slowing which occurs in the AV node. Thus, the ventricular myocardium is activated by two separate pathways (the AP and the AV node), resulting in a fused – or widened – QRS complex. The initial part of the complex, the delta wave, represents aberrant activation of the ventricular myocardium through the AP, while the terminal portion of the QRS represents normal activation through the His-Purkinje system from impulses having traveled through both the AV node and the AP. This classic triad of electrocardiographic findings, when encountered in the setting of a symptomatic dysrhythmia, represents the WPW syndrome. These dysrhythmias include paroxysmal supraventricular tachycardia (also known as AV

reciprocating tachycardia (AVRT)), atrial fibrillation, and ventricular fibrillation.

The most frequently encountered rhythm disturbance is AVRT with two subtypes described; these two subtypes are classified based upon the direction of conduction through the accessory pathway (antegrade versus retrograde) and the resultant QRS complex width. Activation of the ventricular myocardium and impulse propagation occurs either through the AV node or AP. With antegrade conduction through the AV node with impulse return to the atria via the AP, the AVRT is referred to as orthodromic. Orthodromic AVRT, the most common form of AV reciprocating tachycardia, presents electrocardiographically with a narrow QRS complex – and is indistinguishable from typical AV nodal reciprocating tachycardia (i.e. PSVT).

The least common form of AVRT is the antidromic tachycardia, which is seen in approximately 10% of WPW PSVT patients. In this rhythm presentation, the AP conducts the impulse from the atria to the ventricles in antegrade fashion; the impulse returns to the atria via the bundle branches, His-Purkinje fibers and AV node. In this form of AVRT, the QRS complex is wide due to inefficient conduction of the impulse through the ventricular myocardium (i.e. the His-Purkinje system is not used). The QRS complexes appear wide (essentially, an exaggeration of the delta wave) and the ECG displays a very rapid, wide complex tachycardia that is indistinguishable from that of ventricular tachycardia. The ventricular rates are rapid with a range of 180–240 beats/minute. This form of AVRT places the patient at risk for arrhythmic decompensation due to the loss of AV node protection of the ventricle from rapid rates.

The initial treatment of the antidromic AVRT (i.e. the wide complex tachycardia) focuses on interrupting the re-entrant circuit. Electrical cardioversion should be applied to all patients with hemodynamic instability; additionally, tachycardias with ventricular rates approaching 300/minute are at an increased risk of ventricular fibrillation, resulting from myocardial ischemia due to reduced perfusion of the heart as well as

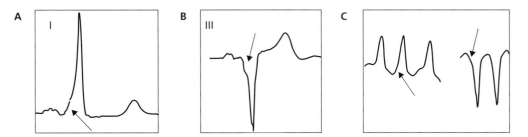

Figure 99.1 A Normal sinus rhythm with PR interval shortening, delta wave (arrow), and widened QRS complex. **B** Normal sinus rhythm with PR interval shortening, delta wave (arrow), and widened QRS complex; note that the delta wave has a negative polarity. **C** Antidromic tachycardia with wide QRS complex; note the initial slurring of the QRS complex which is termed the delta wave (arrow).

subsequent depolarizations falling on the electrically vulnerable repolarization phase. In the hemodynamically stable patient, the agents of first choice would be either procainamide or amiodarone. Agents such as calcium channel antagonists, beta-adrenergic blocking agents, or digoxin which act primarily on the AV node are contraindicated since they will facilitate conduction down the AP and could potentially lead to an increased ventricular rate with ventricular fibrillation.

Further reading

1 Wolff L, Parkinson J, White PD. Bundle-branch block with short PR interval in healthy young people prone to paroxysmal tachycardia. *Am Heart J* 1930;**5**:685–704.

2 Rosner M, Brady WJ, Kefer M, Martin ML. Electrocardiography in the patient with the Wolff–Parkinson–White syndrome: diagnostic and initial therapeutic issues. *Am J Emerg Med* 1999;**17**:705–14.

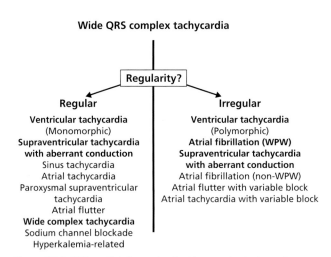

Wide QRS complex tachycardia

Regularity?

Regular
Ventricular tachycardia (Monomorphic)
Supraventricular tachycardia with aberrant conduction
Sinus tachycardia
Atrial tachycardia
Paroxysmal supraventricular tachycardia
Atrial flutter
Wide complex tachycardia
Sodium channel blockade
Hyperkalemia-related

Irregular
Ventricular tachycardia (Polymorphic)
Atrial fibrillation (WPW)
Supraventricular tachycardia with aberrant conduction
Atrial fibrillation (non-WPW)
Atrial flutter with variable block
Atrial tachycardia with variable block

Figure 99.2 Differential diagnosis of wide complex tachycardia.

Case 100 | **Abdominal pain in a trauma victim**

Answer: C

Diagnosis: Splenic rupture

Discussion: The spleen is the most commonly injured intraperitoneal organ after blunt abdominal trauma, followed by the liver and the intestines. Motor vehicle collisions are the most common mechanism of injury (50–75%) in the United States, particularly in children, followed by direct blows to the abdomen (15%) and falls (6–9%). The majority of alert patients will present with abdominal pain or left shoulder pain (Kehr's sign) and have localized left upper quadrant tenderness on exam. Others may exhibit signs of acute intraperitoneal hemorrhage, such as hypotension or tachycardia. Associated risk factors are splenomegaly and substance abuse; only 10–25% of splenic injuries are associated with rib fractures.

In hemodynamically stable patients, abdominal and pelvic computerized axial tomography (CT) imaging can reliably identify solid organ and retroperitoneal pathology after blunt trauma. Using oral contrast rarely increases diagnostic accuracy and simply delays imaging. Although the focused assessment by sonography in trauma (FAST) exam can be used to rapidly detect intraperitoneal blood, it cannot reliably identify injuries to solid organs, the retroperitoneum, or the diaphragm.

Advances in diagnostic imaging have revolutionized the management of splenic injuries. CT imaging can accurately define the degree of splenic disruption such that more injuries are treated nonoperatively. Operative management is dependent on the extent of the injury (Table 100.1). Most recently, up to 90% of children and 50% of adults are treated success-

Table 100.1 American Association for the Surgery of Trauma – Splenic Injury Scale

Grade	Type	Injury	Treatment
I	Hematoma	Subcapsular, <10% surface area (SA)	NO
	Laceration	Capsular tear, <1 cm parenchymal depth	
II	Hematoma	Subcapsular, <50% SA; intraparenchymal, <5 cm diameter	NO
	Laceration	1–3 cm parenchymal depth	
III	Hematoma	Subcapsular, >50% SA; intraparenchymal, >5 cm	NO/O
	Laceration	>3 cm parenchymal depth or involving trabecular vessels	
IV	Laceration	Laceration of segmental or hilar vessels (>25% spleen)	O
	Vascular	Hilar vascular injury that devascularizes the spleen	

NO: Nonoperative; O: Operative.

fully without surgery. After discharge, patients should be on bed rest for 72 hours, limit their physical activity for 6 weeks, and withhold contact sports for 6 months.

Delayed splenic rupture, characterized by abdominal pain and/or signs of internal bleeding that develop after an asymptomatic period of at least 48 hours, occurs in 1% of blunt abdominal trauma. About 50% of patients will present within 1 week of their injury, usually precipitated by minor stress such as twisting or bending. Although uncommon, delayed diagnosis or misdiagnosis may cause significant morbidity and mortality.

Further reading

1 Allen TL, Greenlee RR, Price RR. Delayed splenic rupture presenting as unstable angina pectoris: case report and review of the literature. *J Emerg Med* 2002;**23**(2):165–9.

2 Harbrecht BG. Is anything new in adult blunt splenic trauma? *Am J Surg* 2005;**190**(2):273–8.

Index

Note: Page numbers in italics refer to Case Presentations and Questions, while those in bold refer to Answers, Diagnoses, and Discussion.

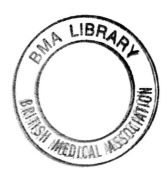